Psychiatry
on the move

Psychiatry
on the move

Authors: **Molly Douglas, Harriet Walker,
Helen Casey**
Editorial Advisor: **Simon Matta**
Series Editors: **Rony Mackinnon, Sally Keat,
Thomas Locke and Andrew Walker**

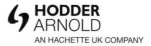
HODDER
ARNOLD
AN HACHETTE UK COMPANY

First published in Great Britain in 2012 by
Hodder Arnold, an imprint of Hodder Education, a division of Hachette UK
338 Euston Road, London NW1 3BH

http://www.hodderarnold.com

British Library Cataloguing in Publication Data
A catalogue record for this book is available from the British Library

Library of Congress Cataloging-in-Publication Data
A catalog record for this book is available from the Library of Congress

ISBN-13   978-1-444-14565-6

1 2 3 4 5 6 7 8 9 10
Commissioning Editor: Joanna Koster
Project Editor: Stephen Clausard
Production Controller: Joanna Walker
Cover Design: Amina Dudhia
Indexer: Laurence Errington

Cover images © Sebastian Kaulitzki – Fotolia & © franckreporter/istockphoto.com (smartphone)

Typeset in 10/12pt Adobe Garamond Pro Regular by Datapage (India) Pvt. Ltd.
Printed and bound in India

> What do you think about this book? Or any other Hodder Arnold title?
> Please visit our website: www.hodderarnold.com

Contents

Preface   xi
List of abbreviations   xiii
An explanation of the text   xvii

PART I: MENTAL HEALTH ASSESSMENT AND
SERVICE PROVISION   1

1. History and mental state examination   3
   1.1   Interview techniques   3
   1.2   Psychiatric history   3
   1.3   The mental state examination   9
   1.4   Risk assessment   15
   1.5   Physical examination in psychiatry   16
   1.6   Relevant investigations   18
   1.7   Summarizing the case   19

2. Mental health and the law   21
   2.1   The Mental Capacity Act   21
   2.2   The Mental Health Act   22

3. The multidisciplinary team approach to psychiatry   24
   3.1   The multidisciplinary team   24
   3.2   Psychiatric services   25
   3.3   Care in the community   26

PART II: MENTAL HEALTH DISORDERS   29

4. Organic mental disorders   33
   4.1   Delirium   33
   4.2   Dementia   38
   4.3   Pseudodementia   42
   4.4   Alzheimer's disease   42
   4.5   Vascular dementia   45
   4.6   Mixed dementia   47
   4.7   Lewy body dementia   47
   4.8   Dementia in Pick's disease (a frontotemporal dementia) 48
   4.9   Old age psychiatry   49
   4.10 Late-onset schizophrenia   49
   4.11 Late-onset bipolar disorder   50
   4.12 Late-onset depressive disorder   51

4.13   Suicide in older people   52
4.14   Substance misuse among older adults   53
4.15   Organic dementia   53
4.16   Head injury   55
4.17   Damage to specific areas of the brain   56
4.18   Endocrine disorders   56
4.19   Metabolic disorders   58
4.20   Nutritional disorders   59
4.21   Autoimmune disorders   60

5. Substance misuse   62
5.1   Assessment of substance misuse   62
5.2   Acute intoxication of alcohol and other substances   64
5.3   Harmful use   66
5.4   Dependence syndrome   67
5.5   Acute withdrawal state   70
5.6   Psychotic disorder associated with substance misuse   70
5.7   Wernicke's encephalopathy and Korsakoff's syndrome   71
5.8   Residual and late-onset psychotic disorder   73
5.9   Other commonly abused substances   74

6. Schizophrenia and delusional disorders   77
6.1   Schizophrenia   77
6.2   Delusional disorders   89
6.3   Acute and transient psychotic disorders   93
6.4   Induced delusional disorder (folie à deux)   96
6.5   Schizoaffective disorders   97

7. Affective disorders   100
7.1   Manic episode   100
7.2   Depressive episode   104
7.3   Recurrent depressive disorder   113
7.4   Bipolar affective disorder   115
7.5   Other affective disorders   119

8. Anxiety and neuroses   123
8.1   Generalized anxiety disorder   123
8.2   Mixed anxiety and depression   125
8.3   Panic disorder   126
8.4   Specific phobia   128
8.5   Agoraphobia   129
8.6   Social phobia   130
8.7   Obsessive–compulsive disorder   132

8.8   Acute stress reaction   134
8.9   Post-traumatic stress disorder   135
8.10   Adjustment disorder   137
8.11   Somatization disorder   138
8.12   Hypochondriacal disorder   139
8.13   Somatoform autonomic dysfunction   140
8.14   Somatoform pain disorder   140

9. Behavioural syndromes associated with physiological
   disturbance   142
   9.1   Eating disorders   142
   9.2   Sleep disorders   147
   9.3   Psychosexual disorders   151
   9.4   Disorders related to the puerperium and menstruation   155

10. Disorders of adult personality   162
    10.1   Definition   162
    10.2   Epidemiology   162
    10.3   Aetiology   162
    10.4   Classification   163
    10.5   Treatment   168
    10.6   Prognosis   169

11. Learning disability and child and adolescent disorders   170
    11.1   General learning disability   170
    11.2   Down's syndrome   174
    11.3   Fragile X syndrome   175
    11.4   Fetal alcohol syndrome   175
    11.5   Psychiatric assessment in children   176
    11.6   Conduct disorders   176
    11.7   Oppositional defiant disorder   178
    11.8   Disorders of social functioning   178
    11.9   Hyperkinetic disorder   179
    11.10 Autism   180
    11.11 Asperger's syndrome   182
    11.12 Tourette's syndrome   183
    11.13 Non-organic enuresis   184
    11.14 Adolescent depression   185
    11.15 Adolescent suicide and deliberate self-harm   186
    11.16 Adolescent substance misuse   187

12. Forensic psychiatry 189
    12.1 Assessment 189
    12.2 Crime and mental health 189
    12.3 Legal competence 191

13. Pharmacotherapy 192
    13.1 Antidepressants 192
    13.2 Antipsychotics 197
    13.3 Mood stabilizers 206
    13.4 Anxiolytics and hypnotics 209

14. Electroconvulsive therapy and psychotherapy 213
    14.1 Electroconvulsive therapy 213
    14.2 Psychotherapy 215

15. Psychiatric emergencies 218
    15.1 Suicide 218
    15.2 Self-harm 221
    15.3 Lithium toxicity 223
    15.4 Neuroleptic malignant syndrome 225
    15.5 Acute dystonic reaction 227
    15.6 Acute alcohol withdrawal state with delirium 228
    15.7 Aggression and agitation 231

PART III: SELF-ASSESSMENT 235

16. Mental health assessment and service provision 237
    Questions 237
    History and examination: EMQs 237
    Mental health and the law: EMQs 238
    Multidisciplinary team: EMQs 239

    Answers 240
    History and examination: EMQs 240
    Mental health and the law: EMQs 241
    Multidisciplinary team: EMQs 242

17. Mental health disorders 243
    Questions 243
    Organic disorders: EMQs 243
    Substance misuse and acute alcohol withdrawal: SBAs 244
    Schizophrenia and delusional disorders: EMQs 244
    Schizophrenia and delusional disorders: SBAs 247
    Mood disorders: EMQs 248
    Mood disorders: SBAs 249

Anxiety: EMQs   249
Anxiety: SBAs   250
Self-harm and suicide: EMQs   251
Self-harm and suicide: SBA   251
Child and adolescent: SBA   252
Eating disorders: EMQs   252
Forensic: SBA   253
Sleep disorders: SBAs   253

Answers   254
Organic disorders: EMQs   254
Substance misuse and acute alcohol withdrawal: SBAs   254
Schizophrenia and delusional disorders: EMQs   255
Schizophrenia and delusional disorders: SBAs   256
Mood disorders: EMQs   257
Mood disorders: SBAs   257
Anxiety: EMQs   258
Anxiety: SBAs   258
Self-harm and suicide: EMQs   259
Self-harm and suicide: SBA   259
Child and adolescent: SBA   259
Eating disorders: EMQs   259
Forensic: SBA   260
Sleep disorders: SBAs   260

18. Treatment and psychiatric emergencies   261

Questions   261
Electroconvulsive therapy and psychotherapy: SBA   261
Lithium and mood stabilizers: SBAs   261
Antidepressants: EMQs   262
Antidepressants: SBA   262
Antipsychotics: EMQs   263
Acute dystonic reaction: SBA   263

Answers   264
Electroconvulsive therapy and psychotherapy: SBA   264
Lithium and mood stabilizers: SBAs   264
Antidepressants: EMQs   264
Antidepressants: SBA   265
Antipsychotics: EMQs   265
Acute dystonic reaction: SBA   265

Index   267

Preface

Have you ever found psychiatry overwhelmingly complicated? Are you simply short of time and have exams looming? If so, this short revision guide will help you. Written by students and junior doctors, this book presents information in a wide range of formats including flow charts, summary tables, authentic images and figures. During the course of writing this book, some of the students among us have now become qualified doctors ourselves.

Although you will find the fundamental basics to psychiatric disorders within this book always remeber to interpret your findings and observations within the context of the individual presented in front of you as well as the results of any subsequent tests requested and individual responses to treatment. Clinical medicine, and in particular psychiatry therefore requires a certain sense of intuition that can only be gained through prior knowledge of the disorders in question. We hope that this book will give a detailed enough overview of the topics to be able to achieve this.

No matter what your learning style, we hope you will find this book appealing and easy to read. We think that this innovative style will help you, the reader, to connect with this often dreaded specialty – helping you learn and understand it (maybe even enjoy it!) while also helping to prepare you for exams and encounters with psychiatric disorders as a junior doctor.

We of course welcome your feedback on how this book measures up and how you feel it could aid your study and work better. Every day is a new learning experience for us all, and let's not forget: medicine is about life-long learning!

AUTHORS

Molly Douglas BMedSci MBChB – Foundation Year 1 doctor, Trafford General Hospital, Manchester, UK
Harriet Walker AVCM (Hons) – Final Year medical student, University of Sheffield, UK
Helen Casey MBChB – Foundation Year 1 doctor, Southmead Hospital, Bristol, UK

EDITORIAL ADVISOR

Simon Matta BSc BMedSci BM BS MSc MRCPsych – Consultant Psychiatrist, Humber NHS Foundation Trust, UK

EDITOR-IN-CHIEF

Rory Mackinnon BSc MBChB – Foundation Year 2 doctor, Northern General Hospital, Sheffield, UK

SERIES EDITORS

Sally Keat BMedSci MBChB – Foundation Year 1 doctor, Northern General Hospital, Sheffield, UK

Thomas Locke BSc MBChB – Foundation Year 1 doctor, Northern General Hospital, Sheffield, UK

Andrew Walker BMedSci MBChB – Specialist Trainee Year 1 doctor in Medicine, Chesterfield Royal Hospital, Chesterfield, Derbyshire, UK

List of abbreviations

- 5-HIAA: 5-hydroxyindoleacetic acid
- 5-HT: 5-hydroxytryptamine (serotonin)
- ABC: airway, breathing and circulation
- ACE: angiotensin-converting enzyme
- ACTH: adrenocorticotropic hormone
- ADHD: attention-deficit hyperactivity disorder
- ADLs: activities of daily living
- ADOS: autism diagnostic observation schedule
- AIDS: acquired immune deficiency syndrome
- ALT: alanine aminotransferase
- AMHP: approved mental health professional
- AMT: abbreviated mental test score
- ApoE: apolipoprotein E
- APP: amyloid precursor protein
- AST: aspartate aminotransferase
- ASW: approved social worker
- BAD: bipolar affective disorder
- BMI: body mass index
- BNF: *British National Formulary*
- BP: blood pressure
- CAGE: four-part series of questions used to assess an individual's level of addiction to alcohol
- CAM: confusion assessment method
- CAT: cognitive analytical therapy
- CBM: cognitive bias model
- CBT: cognitive behavioural therapy
- CCBT: computerized cognitive behavioural therapy
- CD: conduct disorder
- CDM: cognitive deficit model
- CJD: Creutzfeldt–Jakob disease
- CMHT: community mental health team
- CMV: cytomegalovirus
- CNS: central nervous system
- COCP: combined oral contraceptive pill
- COPD: chronic obstructive pulmonary disease
- CPA: care programme approach
- CPN: community psychiatric nurse
- CRF: corticotrophin releasing factor
- CRP: C-reactive protein

- CT: computed tomography
- CTPA: computed tomography pulmonary angiogram
- CVA: cerebrovascular accident
- DEXA: dual energy X-ray absorptiometry
- DBT: dialectical behavioural therapy
- D.O.B.: date of birth
- DST: dexamethasone suppression test
- DT: delirium tremens
- ECG: electrocardiogram
- ECT: electroconvulsive therapy
- ED: emergency department
- EEG: electroencephalogram
- eGFR: estimated glomerular filtration rate
- EMDR: eye movement desensitization and reprogramming
- EPDS: Edinburgh Postnatal Depression Scale
- EPSE: extrapyramidal side-effects
- FBC: full blood count
- FSH: follicle-stimulating hormone
- FTD: formal thought disorder
- GABA: gamma-aminobutyric acid
- GAD: generalized anxiety disorder
- GCS: Glasgow coma scale
- GDS: geriatric depression scale
- GGT: gamma-glutamyltransferase
- GH: growth hormone
- GP: general practitioner
- HAART: highly active anti-retroviral therapy
- HIV: human immunodeficiency virus
- ICU: intensive care unit
- IM: intramuscular
- INR: international normalized ratio
- IPT: interpersonal therapy
- IV: intravenous
- IVDU: intravenous drug user
- LDL: low-density lipoprotein
- LFTs: liver function tests
- LH: luteinizing hormone
- LSD: lysergic acid diethylamide
- MAO: monoamine oxidase
- MAOIs: monoamine oxidase inhibitors
- MDT: multidisciplinary team
- MHA: Mental Health Act
- MI: myocardial infarction

- MMSE: mini-mental state examination
- MRI: magnetic resonance imaging
- MSE: mental state examination
- MSU: mid-stream urine
- NHS: National Health Service
- NICE: National Institute for Health and Clinical Excellence
- NMDA: N-methyl-D-aspartate
- NMS: neuroleptic malignant syndrome
- NSAIDs: non-steroidal anti-inflammatory drugs
- OCD: obsessive–compulsive disorder
- ODD: oppositional defiant disorder
- OSA: obstructive sleep apnoea
- PD: personality disorder
- PDE5: phosphodiesterase type 5 inhibitors
- PE: pulmonary embolism
- PHQ-9: Patient Health Questionnaire
- PMS: premenstrual syndrome
- PO: oral administration (per os)
- PPHN: persistent pulmonary hypertension of the newborn
- PTH: parathyroid hormone
- PTSD: post-traumatic stress disorder
- QTc: corrected QT interval
- RC: responsible clinician
- REM: rapid eye movement
- SaO_2: oxygen saturation
- SCT: supervised community treatment
- SLE: systemic lupus erythematosus
- SSRI: selective serotonin re-uptake inhibitor
- STR: support time and recovery
- T_3: triiodothyronine
- T_4: thyroxine
- TCA: tricyclic antidepressant
- TDS: to be taken three times daily
- TENS: transcutaneous electrical nerve stimulation
- TFTs: thyroid function tests
- TIA: transient ischaemic attack
- TSH: thyroid-stimulating hormone
- U&E: urea and electrolytes
- UTI: urinary tract infection
- VDRL: Venereal Disease Research Laboratory
- Y-BOCS: Yale-Brown Obsessive Compulsive Scale

An explanation of the text

The book is divided into three parts: mental health assessment and service provision, mental health disorders and a self-assessment section. We have used bullet points to keep the text concise and brief and supplemented this with a range of diagrams, pictures, tables and MICRO-boxes (explained below).

MICRO-facts

These boxes expand on the text and contain clinically relevant facts and memorable summaries of the essential information.

MICRO-print

These boxes contain additional information to the text that may interest certain readers but is not essential for everybody to learn.

MICRO-case

These boxes contain clinical cases relevant to the text and include a number of summary bullet points to highlight the key learning objectives.

MICRO-references

These boxes contain references to important clinical research and national guidance.

Normal range values are given for most tests in this book as a guideline for your knowledge. Please note that ranges differ between laboratories and therefore you should always use figures from your own institution to interpret results.

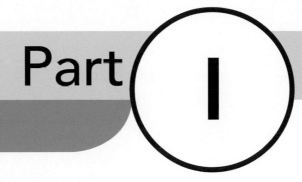

Part 1

Mental health assessment and service provision

1. History and mental state examination   3
   1.1   Interview techniques   3
   1.2   Psychiatric history   3
   1.3   The mental state examination   9
   1.4   Risk assessment   15
   1.5   Physical examination in psychiatry   17
   1.6   Relevant investigations   17
   1.7   Summarizing the case   19

2. Mental health and the law   21
   2.1   The Mental Capacity Act   21
   2.2   The Mental Health Act   22

3. The multidisciplinary team approach to psychiatry   24
   3.1   The multidisciplinary team   24
   3.2   Psychiatric services   25
   3.3   Care in the community   26

1 History and mental state examination

1.1 INTERVIEW TECHNIQUES

- **Open questions:** *'Can you tell me why you were admitted?'* Open-ended questions are often used in the initial phase of the interview to produce spontaneous responses from the patient, which are potentially what feels most important to the patient. They convey a sense of genuine interest to the patient.
- **Closed questions:** *'Did you attempt to end your life prior to admission?'* Closed-ended questions often follow open-ended questions to efficiently elicit specific details.
- **Summation (summarizing)** refers to the brief summary of what the person has said so far and is done periodically to ensure that the interviewer understands the person correctly: e.g. *'I would like to make sure that I understand you correctly so far. You are saying that you do not think your experience is part of schizophrenia based on your own readings'* (to a man who does not believe that he suffers from schizophrenia and wants to seek a second opinion).
- **Empathic statements** convey the message that the psychiatrist finds the patient's concern important and acknowledges the patient's sufferings: e.g. *'I can imagine that you were terrified when you realized that you could not move half of your body'* (to a man suffering from post-stroke depression).

1.2 PSYCHIATRIC HISTORY

DEMOGRAPHICS

Similar to history taking in other specialties, some basic information about the patient is required:
- name;
- age/date of birth (D.O.B.);
- sex;
- current occupation;
- marital status;

- route of referral (e.g. general practice, emergency department (ED)) and reason for referral;
- setting of the psychiatric interview (e.g. outpatient clinic, ward);
- details of any informants present and their relationship to the patient.

PRESENTING COMPLAINT

- Document the patient's views on why he was referred/admitted in his own words as far as possible.
- List all symptoms:
  - try to group symptoms if they fall naturally in a diagnostic category, e.g. group lack of motivation, reduced energy and insomnia as these are all depressive symptoms;
  - list symptoms (or groups of symptoms) in order of decreasing severity (most distressing and severe first).

HISTORY OF PRESENTING COMPLAINT

A systematic approach should be taken for each presenting complaint that the patient has, and the patient's own words used as far as possible. A useful approach is as follows:

- Nature of the complaint:
  - list all symptoms chronologically with the most recent symptoms listed last – this will help characterize the evolution of the illness(es).
- Describe any important negatives (symptoms or signs that could have been expected but were not present; e.g. no thought interference phenomena in a psychotic patient).
- Establish the onset, duration, patterns and chronicity of all presenting complaints:
  - are they longstanding problems or have they occurred more acutely?
  - is there a relapsing, remitting pattern?
  - when was the patient last well?
- Any precipitating factors or triggers?
- Explore how the problem is affecting their relationships and social functioning; e.g. are they able to work?
- Aggravating and relieving factors.
- Any similar previous episodes?
- Is there a temporal relationship with physical/psychological or social problems?
- If required, try to get a collateral history from family members, etc.
- Include any treatments received so far (current episode) describing effects and side-effects if any.

Mental health assessment and service provision

PAST PSYCHIATRIC HISTORY

Has the patient suffered with any psychiatric problems in the past, with specific details including:
- previous diagnoses;
- duration of symptoms;
- treatments, including drug dose, effects and side-effects;
- any previous treatments using psychological interventions;
- information about inpatient, day hospital and outpatient care;
- any compulsory admissions or treatment;
- any history of deliberate self-harm;
- any current medications being taken.

PAST MEDICAL AND SURGICAL HISTORY

- Any medical problems currently or in the past (in particular chronic pain, seizures (e.g. temporal lobe epilepsy), stroke, head injury, endocrine disorders (e.g. thyroid disorders) and heart diseases).
- Have they had any surgery?
- Are they being treated by their general practitioner (GP) for anything?

MEDICATION HISTORY AND ALLERGIES

Include medications that they have been prescribed for any psychiatric problems and for any other illnesses. Include:
- drug name;
- dose;
- duration;
- therapeutic benefit;
- any adverse reactions;
- past drug history and reasons for stopping them;
- allergies:
  - drugs:
    - what happens when you take this drug?
  - any non-drug products (e.g. foods or latex).

FAMILY HISTORY AND FAMILY PSYCHIATRIC HISTORY

Information should be obtained about:
- The patient's parents and the relationships they have with them.
- Any siblings and the relationships that they have with them.
- Note the occupation and ages of all family members if possible.
- Note the cause (e.g. suicide) and age of death of deceased family members.
- It may be helpful to draw a family tree similar to the one shown in Fig. 1.1.

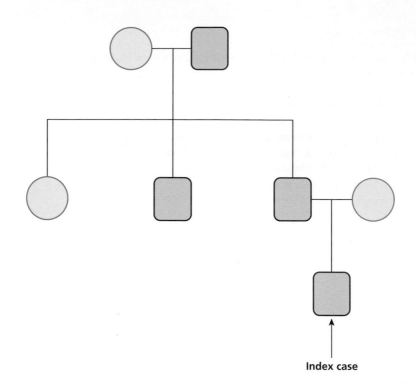

Index case

Fig. 1.1 Example of a family tree.

Specifically, ask about any mental illness within the family and any other familial illnesses.

PERSONAL HISTORY

This section needs to be split into four distinct areas. These are: developmental history, educational history, employment history and relationships.

- Developmental history:
  - pregnancy and birth – any complications and mode of delivery?
  - did they reach developmental milestones?
  - any health problems as a child?
  - family environment:
    - any emotional, physical or sexual abuse?
    - separations or bereavements in childhood,
    - most importantly, was it a happy childhood?
  - childhood home environment, e.g. living conditions, deprivation.
- Educational history:
  - details of schooling – age that schooling began and stopped;
  - truancy or bullying;

- academic achievements:
    - any GCSEs, A Levels, degrees or postgraduate qualifications?
- relationships with peers (friendship groups, social isolation).
- Employment history:
    - are they currently working?
    - chronological list of jobs:
        - job titles,
        - duration,
        - reason for changing jobs;
    - work satisfaction;
    - relationships with colleagues.
- Relationships:
    - sexual orientation;
    - chronological list of all major relationships/marriages;
    - reasons for relationship breakdown;
    - any abuse?
    - if in a current relationship:
        - is the partner supportive?
        - is there good communication?
        - any infidelity?
- Any children?
    - Who do they live with?
    - What is the relationship like?
- For women only:
    - age of onset of menarche;
    - menstrual pattern;
    - contraception;
    - miscarriages, stillbirths and any terminations.

SOCIAL HISTORY

- Where does the patient currently live and with whom?
- Financial details: working or on benefits?
- Daily activities and hobbies.
- Details of support network.
- Religion.
- Comment on relationship with others, e.g. neighbours if appropriate.
- Any safety and vulnerability issues?
- Any child protection issues?

Mental health assessment and service provision

DRUGS AND ALCOHOL HISTORY

- Which drugs?/amounts used?/route?
- Effects/side-effects.
- Financial aspects (how is the habit funded?).
- Complications (physical, forensic, psychological).
- History of treatments (e.g. admission for planned alcohol detox).
- Alcohol – CAGE, dependence questions.

MICRO-facts

CAGE questions

Have you ever:

- felt you should **C**ut down on your drinking?
- been **A**nnoyed by others criticising your drinking?
- felt bad or **G**uilty about your drinking?
- had a drink first thing in the morning to steady your nerves (**E**ye-opener)?

- Use of tobacco.

More details about taking an alcohol and drug history can be found in Chapter 5 Substance misuse, Assessment of substance misuse.

PREMORBID PERSONALITY

A good collateral history would greatly enhance assessment of premorbid personality.

- How would they describe themselves?
- How do they think others would describe their personality?
- Has this changed since they became unwell?
- Relationships/friendships:
  - few/many;
  - superficial/close.
- Attitude towards own and the opposite sex.
- Attitude towards colleagues and superiors.
- Hobbies and interests.
- Predominant mood/emotions (e.g. anxious, overconfident).
- Character traits (e.g. impulsive, perfectionist).
- Attitudes and standards.

FORENSIC HISTORY

- Nature of offence.
- Consequence – caution, charged, custodial sentence?

- Patient's view on incidents.
- Remorse.
- Risk of re-offending.
- Seek collateral information where appropriate.

1.3 THE MENTAL STATE EXAMINATION

The mental state examination (MSE) is an essential part of a psychiatric assessment. It is an exploration of **current symptomatology** and is used to determine whether there is evidence of any mental illness, and if so the severity of the symptoms that the patient is experiencing.

APPEARANCE AND BEHAVIOURS

- Appearance:
    - general appearance and racial origin;
    - facial appearance;
    - self-neglect;
    - style of dress;
    - abnormal involuntary movements.

MICRO-print
Abnormal involuntary movements

Ambitendency – series of tentative and incomplete movements.
Echopraxia – automatic imitation of another person's movements.
Mannerisms – repeated involuntary movements that appear to be goal directed.
Posturing – inappropriate/bizarre bodily postures held continuously for long periods.
Stereotypies – repeated movements that are not goal directed.

- Behaviours:
    - is their behaviour appropriate for the situation?
    - level of motor activity;
    - eye contact;
    - rapport;
    - aggression;
    - distractibility – do they appear to be responding to hallucinations?

SPEECH

- Tone:
    - variations in pitch – may be reduced in depression;
    - loss of tone is seen in chronic psychotic illness and Aspergers syndrome.

- Volume:
  - loud or a whisper.
- Rate:
  - increased rate, volume and pressure of speech is seen in mania.
- Quantity and fluency:
  - how much do they speak and is it fluent? (in poverty of speech there is a restricted amount);
  - stuttering or slurring of speech;
  - echolalia refers to the repetition of words or phrases spoken by another person.
- Form:
  - abnormalities in the FORM of speech are known as formal thought disorder (FTD);
  - there are many different types of FTD. Some of the main ones are shown in Fig. 1.2.

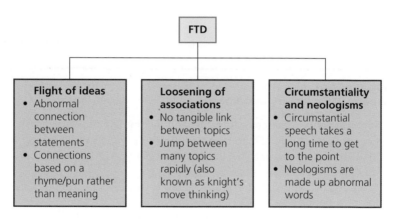

Fig. 1.2 Types of formal thought disorder (FTD).

MOOD AND AFFECT

Mood refers to the pervasive or prevailing emotional state.

- Subjective mood:
  - How the patient says he feels, in his own words;
  - Alexithymia refers to difficulty in understanding or verbalizing one's emotions.
- Objective mood:
  - your description as an assessor:
    - dysphoric mood – an unpleasant mood,
    - euthymic – neither depressed nor elevated mood,

- elated – high mood and exaggerated feelings of well-being (seen in mania).
- apathy – loss of emotion.
- Any fluctuations in mood? – more or less so than normal?
- Incongruent – is the patient's mood inconsistent with their thoughts and feelings?
  - e.g. talking about a bereavement but laughing.

MICRO-facts

A good tip is to get the patient to rate their mood on a scale of 1 to 10, stating clearly what the numbers mean, e.g. 10 = best-ever mood. It is also useful to ask them to rate what their mood is like normally on the same scale.

Affect is the observed external manifestation of the mood/emotion and describes mood at a specific point in time (e.g. at the time of the assessment). It can be described as follows:

- Inappropriate affect: incongruent with the subject being discussed (similar to incongruent mood).
- Blunted affect: lack of a normal emotional response or a reduction in variation in mood and emotions.
- Flat affect: total or almost total absence of reactivity of affect.
- Labile affect: excessively changing affect (increased variation).

PERCEPTION

Definitions:
- Perception: cognitive processing and interpretation of data arriving via the sense organs.
- Illusions:
  - the false perception of a real external stimulus (e.g. thinking that a dressing gown tie is a snake):
    - affect illusions – occur when emotions are increased,
    - completion illusions – the brain's tendency to 'fill-in' the missing part of an object to make it appear meaningful,
    - pareidolic illusions – the tendency to interpret random or ambiguous stimuli and 'see' meaningful images, especially faces and people, when none actually exists (e.g. 'seeing' faces in clouds).
- Hallucinations:
  - a false sensory perception in the absence of a real external stimulus:
    - auditory – frequently seen in psychosis and are discussed in detail in Chapter 6 Schizophrenia and delusional disorders, Schizophrenia.
    - visual – associated with organic disorders of the brain, drug and alcohol withdrawal and are not commonly seen in psychosis,

- olfactory and gustatory (often unpleasant tastes and smells) – rare but can occur in schizophrenia and depression; they can also be indicative of temporal lobe involvement (e.g. temporal lobe epilepsy) or lesions affecting the olfactory pathways,
- tactile/haptic hallucinations: the experience of being touched (e.g. in schizophrenia) or for example, of insects crawling under the skin (e.g. in cocaine users),
- hypnagogic – false perceptions that occur when falling asleep,
- hypnopompic – false perceptions that occur when waking up,
- pseudo-hallucinations – internal perceptions but there is retained insight, i.e. the individual recognizes that the experience originated in their minds not the external world and was not real.

> **MICRO-print**
> Hypnagogic and hypnopompic hallucinations (visual or auditory) frequently occur in completely healthy individuals.

DISORDERS OF THOUGHT

- Thought content:
  - preoccupations:
    - morbid thoughts,
    - patient's main worries,
    - ruminations (recurrent worries that may have a theme) – may occur in anxiety or depression.
- Obsessions:
  - repetitive senseless thoughts that the patient does recognize as his own and as irrational;
  - inability to resist the thoughts.

> **MICRO-print**
> Obsessive thoughts are often followed by compulsive acts as seen in obsessive–compulsive disorder, for example:
> - obsessive thought: 'My mother will come to harm unless I touch the light switch five times.'
> - compulsive act: touch the light switch five times.

- Phobias:
  - ask about any particular phobias, e.g. agoraphobia (fear of crowds, social situations; see Chapter 8 Anxiety and neuroses, Specific phobia, Agoraphobia and Social phobia).

- Abnormal beliefs:
  - overvalued ideas:
    - this is a reasonable and comprehensible idea that is held by the patient but which is pursued beyond normal boundaries and causes distress to the patient [e.g. a young girl of normal body mass index (BMI) believes she is fat but the belief can be challenged].
- Delusions:
  - this is a belief that is held which is fixed, usually false and not in keeping with the educational and cultural background of the patient, and which remains unshakeable even when provided with evidence to the contrary;
  - delusions are classified into primary and secondary:
    - a primary delusion arises out of the blue with no explanation (for example, a schizophrenic man suddenly believes that he is an alien from Mars),
    - a secondary delusion is a consequence of other psychopathology such as auditory hallucination in schizophrenia or grandiosity in mania (for example, a manic patient believes that he is the prime minister of the UK);
  - there are many different types of delusions. The main ones are summarized in Table 1.1.

Table 1.1 Main types of delusions.

TYPE OF DELUSION	CONTENT OF DELUSION
Persecutory	The patient believes that others are out to cause them harm or kill them (e.g. 'Terrorists are trying to kill me')
Nihilistic	Other people, part of their bodies, themselves or the world do not exist or are about to cease to exist (e.g. 'I am already dead, nothing around me is really there anymore')
Of reference	The actions of other people, events, media, etc., are referring to the person (e.g. 'I get special messages from the TV, they talk directly to me and about me in the News')
Of poverty	The patient believes they are in extreme poverty although they are not (e.g. 'I do not have anything at all, no house, no job, no money')
Grandiose	The exaggerated belief of their own power and importance (e.g. 'I am able to heal people just by touching them once')
Of jealousy	The patient is jealous or suspects their partner of being unfaithful without any evidence (e.g. 'I know she is cheating on me because she keeps wearing red')

- Passivity phenomenon (delusion of control):
  - actions, feelings or impulses can be controlled or interfered with by an external agent or force.
- Thought alienation (delusion with regards to the possession of thoughts):
  - **thought insertion**: the belief that thoughts are being put into your head by an external force/person/agent;
  - **thought withdrawal**: the belief that your thoughts are being taken out of your head by an external force/person/agent;
  - **thought broadcast**: the belief that your thoughts are being broadcast out loud for everyone around to hear.

COGNITION

- Orientation:
  - are they orientated to time (day, date, time), place and person?
- Attention and concentration:

> **MICRO-facts**
>
> Attention – the ability of a person to maintain his or her conscious awareness on an external stimulus and to screen out irrelevant stimuli. Concentration – refers to sustained and focused attention.

  - can they spell the word 'WORLD' backwards? or
  - can they do the serial 7s test? (i.e. subtract 7 from 100, then subtract 7 from the remainder, and so on).
- Memory:
  - long- and short-term memory should be assessed as well as immediate recall;
  - if the patient is aged over 65 years or shows evidence of cognitive impairment then more formal testing should be done, e.g. mini-mental state examination (MMSE).

INSIGHT

This is a means of assessing the level of understanding the patient has about their symptoms/illness. Questions can be asked to determine how much insight the patient has.

- Do you think that you are ill?
- Do you accept that your condition is caused by a psychiatric illness?
- Do you accept psychiatric treatment?
  You can use the answers to these three questions to report the level of insight that the patient has.

EXAMPLE CASE

An example case is given below to demonstrate how to report the mental state examination.

MICRO-case

Appearance and behaviours: Mr X is a 38-year-old man who is dressed appropriately with some evidence of self-neglect. He decides to lie on the examination couch rather than sit in the chair. Eye contact was variable.

Speech and thought form: normal tone, rate and volume. Evidence of loosening of associations, particularly tangential speech.

Mood: objectively euthymic, subjectively 'OK'. Affect was reactive.

Thought content: evidence of persecutory delusions – 'Lucifer brought me onto the ward to get rid of me. The police, the government, everybody is trying to get me. They are all devils.'

Perceptions: experiences second-person auditory hallucinations of a persecutory nature: e.g. I hear a voice telling me 'I'm going to smash your head in and kill you'.

Cognition: not orientated to time, person or place. More formal assessment should be carried out.

Insight: partial, as he is aware that 'something is not right' and is willing to accept treatment.

1.4 RISK ASSESSMENT

This is an important part of every complete psychiatric assessment. For ease it can be thought of in three separate parts: risk of harm to self, risk of harm to others and risk of harm from others.

RISK OF SELF-HARM

More information on assessing the suicidal patient can be found in Chapter 15 Psychiatric emergencies, Suicide. Here are some important questions that can be asked:

- Do you have any thoughts of harming yourself/ending your life?
- If yes, do you have any plans?
- Do you think that you would be able to go through with it?
- Have you sorted out your personal affairs?
- Are there any protective factors (e.g. partner or children)?
- Have there been any attempts to harm yourself in the past?
  - take details about each event.

RISK OF HARM TO OTHERS

You will have taken a forensic history earlier, but even if there are no apparent forensic issues, in this section you must still ask:

- Do they have any thoughts or intentions to harm others?
- Any history of violence?
    - document details of dates, nature, severity, etc.
- Do they have any history of arson?
- Have there been any acts of sexually inappropriate behaviour?

As for risk of self-harm you should investigate the protective factors and risk factors and use these in combination with the answers to the above questions to determine the risk to others.

RISK OF HARM FROM OTHERS AND SELF-NEGLECT

- How are they functioning at home?
- Are they managing to complete their activities of daily living?
- Has the situation changed since they became unwell?
- If there appear to be areas that the patient is likely to struggle with, appropriate help and support can be arranged.

These individuals may also be vulnerable to abuse from others. This is harder to assess directly but, having taken a detailed history you should be able to make a decision as to whether your patient is likely to be at risk or vulnerable in their current state.

MICRO-facts

Hyperkinetic disorder – need to assess the risk of accidents resulting from poor impulse control and hyperactivities.

Cognitive impairment – in the elderly, need to assess the risk of fall, fire, accidents and exploitation.

1.5 PHYSICAL EXAMINATION IN PSYCHIATRY

It is essential that all patients have a thorough physical examination because:

- Physical illness may be a consequence of psychiatric illness.
- Psychiatric drugs may cause physical side-effects.
- Physical illness can present with psychiatric symptoms such as delirium.
- There may be an associated physical illness that needs treatment.

- It is important to know the physical health of your patient as well as their mental health at presentation.

    The main areas to address when carrying out a full examination include:
- general appearance/condition;
- cardiovascular;
- respiratory;
- abdominal;
- neurological.

    Figs. 1.3, 1.4 and 1.5 list some key areas to look out for in the physical examination of patients with certain psychiatric conditions.

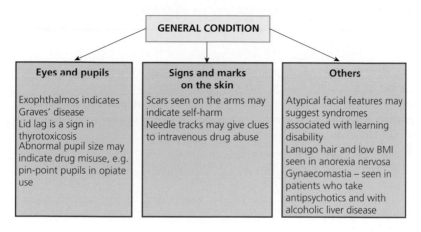

Fig. 1.3 General signs to look for in a psychiatric patient. BMI, body mass index.

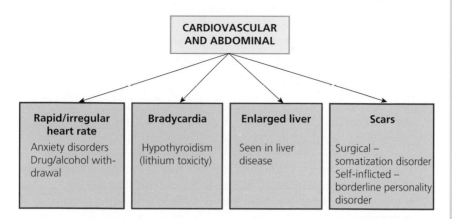

Fig. 1.4 Cardiovascular and abdominal signs to look for in a psychiatric patient.

Mental health assessment and service provision

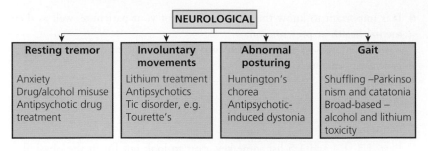

Fig. 1.5 Neurological signs to look for in a psychiatric patient.

1.6 RELEVANT INVESTIGATIONS

BLOOD TESTS

You must check for an organic cause of the symptoms (see Chapter 4) that the patient is presenting with so that one is not missed. It is important to rule out any organic cause for a psychiatric presentation. Routine blood tests also provide a baseline against which to assess the effects of new treatments:

- full blood count (FBC);
- urea and electrolytes (U&E);
- thyroid function tests (TFTs);
- liver function tests (LFTs);
- vitamin B_{12} and folate levels (if you suspect drug and/or alcohol misuse);
- syphilis serology.

URINARY TESTS

This is useful in the following circumstances:

- suspected drug misuse;
- a patient presenting with delirium and you are looking for a cause of infection; this is particularly important in the elderly.

ELECTROCARDIOGRAM

- This is useful in patients who are prescribed antipsychotics. Antipsychotics may prolong the QTc (>430 ms in men and >450 ms in women).

NEUROLOGICAL INVESTIGATIONS

- Electroencephalogram (EEG) and methods such as computed tomography (CT) or magnetic resonance imaging (MRI) are useful to rule out neurological causes (e.g. epilepsy, stroke or brain tumour) of psychiatric symptoms.

1.7 SUMMARIZING THE CASE

The psychiatric case should be reported in a systematic and concise manner as, potentially, there is a lot of information to feedback to your seniors. A helpful way of doing this is to provide a case summary. However, when reporting in the notes it is important to split the case into its different sections:
- history (broken down into the relevant sections);
- mental state examination (broken down into the relevant sections);
- physical examination findings;
- case summary.

The case summary is important as it is a means of providing the most important findings from the history and examination.

CASE SUMMARY

- Synopsis of the history:
  - this would include a brief background about the patient and the salient points from the history incorporating information about:
    - personal information,
    - presenting symptoms and presentation,
    - previous psychiatric illness,
    - risk assessment,
    - positive findings on the mental state examination,
    - insight.
- Differential diagnosis:
  - this gives you the opportunity to formulate a list of differential diagnoses that are likely to fit with the presenting problem;
  - it is worth thinking about the hierarchical pyramid of differential diagnoses shown in Fig. 1.6:
    - you should work from the top down when making a diagnosis to ensure that all organic/medical causes are excluded before making a psychiatric diagnosis.
- Formulation:
  - the 'three Ps':
    - predisposing factors – risk factors that will make it more likely to develop a certain condition,
    - precipitating factors – events/circumstances that led to the onset of the condition,
    - perpetuating factors – factors that are ongoing and, while present, are likely to keep the patient in the mental state that they are in.
  - This helps to clarify why the patient might have become ill and why specifically at this point in time.

Mental health assessment and service provision

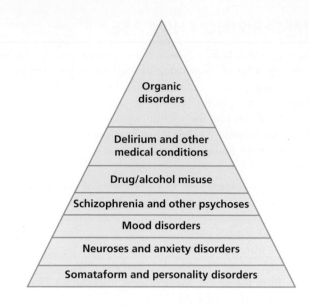

Fig. 1.6 Hierarchy of psychiatric differential diagnoses.

- Management plan:
    - the 'three Ps' will guide your management plan;
    - split into immediate and long term;
    - include the relevant investigations that you will carry out;
    - immediate treatment;
    - long-term treatment;
    - it is important to share information with the rest of the team including information about:
        - risk assessment,
        - is the patient detainable under the Mental Health Act?

2 Mental health and the law

2.1 THE MENTAL CAPACITY ACT

WHAT IS CAPACITY?

- The mental ability to make a decision.
- It depends on the ability to:
  - **understand** the information important to making the decision;
  - **retain** the information for long enough to make the decision;
  - **use or weigh** that information as part of the process of making the decision;
  - **communicate** the decision (by talking or any other means, e.g. sign language).
- It is specific to the time of the decision and the decision itself:
  - a person may be able to make decisions about what they want to wear but not decisions about handling their finances;
  - a person may be capable of making decisions then get ill and not be capable. When they have recovered they will be able to make decisions as before.

LACKING CAPACITY

- A person may lack capacity if, at the time of the decision, they have an impairment of, or a disturbance in the functioning of, the mind or the brain.
- This may be permanent (in advanced dementia) or temporary (a patient with delirium).
- A person who is detained under the Mental Health Act (MHA) may still have capacity to make decisions, although they are not allowed to refuse treatment for their psychiatric problem.

ASSESSING CAPACITY

- A person must be assumed to have capacity until assessed otherwise.
- All practical steps must be taken to maximize a person's ability to make decisions.
- People are allowed to make unwise decisions: this is not an indicator of lack of capacity.

- The decision must be taken in the person's best interest.
- If a decision is made for someone it should be the least restrictive option with regard to their rights and freedom.

2.2 THE MENTAL HEALTH ACT

DEFINITIONS

- Mental disorder is defined as 'any disorder or disability of mind'.
- Patients can be detained ('sectioned') under the MHA if:
  - they have a mental disorder;
  - they pose a risk to themselves or others;
  - they require treatment but refuse informal admission;
  - they do not have insight and refuse necessary treatment.
- Unless otherwise specified, medical recommendations for detention under the MHA require that at least one doctor must be approved under Section 12(2) as a clinician with experience in the diagnosis and treatment of mental disorder.

SECTION 2: ADMISSION FOR ASSESSMENT

- Duration: 28 days maximum.
- Application by: nearest relative or approved mental health professional (AMHP).
- Procedure: two doctors must confirm that the patient appears to be suffering from a mental disorder that warrants assessment.

SECTION 3: ADMISSION FOR TREATMENT

- Duration: up to 6 months, renewable for another 6 months then 1 year or more if necessary.
- Application by: nearest relative or AMHP.
- Procedure: two doctors must confirm that the patient suffers from a mental disorder, appropriate treatment is available and that it is necessary that they are detained in hospital to receive this treatment.

SECTION 4: ADMISSION FOR ASSESSMENT IN EMERGENCY

- Duration: 72 hours maximum.
- Application by: nearest relative or AMHP (who must have seen the patient in the previous 24 hours).
- Procedure: one doctor must confirm that it is urgent the patient be detained.

SECTION 5(2): COMPULSORY DETENTION OF A PSYCHIATRIC PATIENT ALREADY IN HOSPITAL VOLUNTARILY

- Duration: 72 hours maximum.

- Application by: doctor in charge of patient's informal treatment for a mental or physical problem (this can be any doctor).
- Procedure: can detain a patient by reporting to hospital managers that an application for admission should be made.
- This **cannot** be used in an emergency department as it is not an inpatient unit.

SUPERVISED COMMUNITY TREATMENT

- Supervised community treatments (SCTs) are appropriate for patients that:
  - were previously admitted under Section 3;
  - are deemed well enough by their responsible clinician (RC) to leave hospital;
  - remain at risk of disengaging from treatment;
  - may need to be admitted to hospital again at short notice.
- A SCT means a patient can be recalled to hospital for treatment if the RC believes it is necessary.

3 The multidisciplinary team approach to psychiatry

3.1 THE MULTIDISCIPLINARY TEAM

THE TEAM

The multidisciplinary team (MDT) includes:
- psychiatrist;
- psychiatric nurse;
- community psychiatric nurse;
- social worker;
- clinical psychologist;
- secretary/administrator;
- occupational therapist;
- pharmacist.

Some teams may have additional members such as:
- housing advisors;
- support time and recovery (STR) workers;
- physiotherapists.

ROLES OF TEAM MEMBERS

- Psychiatrist:
  - to assess and diagnose mental illness;
  - decision-making on management;
  - prescribing and monitoring of medication;
  - management of physical health problems;
  - decision-making regarding detaining patients under the Mental Health Act (MHA).
- Psychiatric nurse (inpatient):
  - routine nursing care of inpatients;
  - observation and monitoring of inpatients' mental state;
  - administer medication;
  - ensure patient safety (close observations of high-risk patients; de-escalate risky situations involving agitated patients; control and restraint of aggressive patients);
  - therapeutic interventions through one-to-one sessions.

- Community psychiatric nurse:
  - assessment and monitoring of the patient in the community;
  - administer medication;
  - some community psychiatric nurses (CPNs) may have additional skills (e.g. cognitive behavioural therapy).
- Social worker:
  - assesses social circumstances;
  - assistance with accommodation and benefits;
  - approved mental health professionals (AMHPs), previously known as approved social workers (ASWs), are involved in the assessment and detention of patients under the MHA;
  - aid in cases where there are child protection issues or vulnerable adults.
- Clinical psychologist:
  - assessment for psychological treatment;
  - provide psychological treatments (e.g. cognitive behavioural therapy).
- Secretary/administrator:
  - general administrative duties including the organization and coordination of meetings.
- Occupational therapist:
  - assessment and management of daily functioning and independence;
  - assisting with attendance at courses to obtain skills to return to work;
  - provide activities such as art and pottery for inpatients;
  - assist other members of the MDT, such as nursing staff, in the running of healthy living (smoking cessation, healthy diet, etc.) and physical exercise groups.
- Pharmacist:
  - advice and assistance on pharmacological management.

3.2 PSYCHIATRIC SERVICES

There are many services available to psychiatric patients both as an inpatient and in the community.
- Self-help:
  - support groups;
  - manuals.
- Criminal justice system:
  - probation services;
  - prison mental health teams.
- Local authority services:
  - accommodation services/housing;
  - benefit system.

Mental health assessment and service provision

- Crisis team:
  - specialist team available in times of mental health crisis;
  - home visits and increased support.
- Psychiatric hospital:
  - inpatient services;
  - day centre.
- Community mental health teams:
  - support within the community;
  - input from all members of the MDT (see later under Care in the community).
- General hospital:
  - accident and emergency services;
  - liaison psychiatrist;
  - outpatient appointments.
- Primary care:
  - general practitioner (GP);
  - practice nurse.

3.3 CARE IN THE COMMUNITY

THE COMMUNITY MENTAL HEALTH TEAM

- Community psychiatrist.
- Community psychiatric nurses.
- Social workers.
- Occupational therapists.
- Psychologists.

> **MICRO-print**
> There are specialized community mental health teams (CMHTs) for certain age groups. These are:
> - child and adolescent <18 years;
> - general adult 18–65 years;
> - older adults >65 years.

SPECIALIST TEAMS

- Crisis resolution and home treatment teams:
  - provide intensive support for patients in crisis in their own homes;
  - operates 24 hours a day;
  - can see patients more than once a day;
  - help to reduce hospital admissions and support early discharge.

- Assertive outreach teams:
  - provide intensive support and treatment for complex and high-need patients in the community;
  - for patients who are chronically unwell;
  - help with individuals who are at high risk of disengaging with services.
- Early intervention in psychosis services:
  - for patients who are newly diagnosed with psychosis;
  - intensive treatment for the first 2–3 years of illness;
  - aim to promote early recovery from the illness.

THE CARE COORDINATOR AND THE CARE PROGRAMME APPROACH

The management of individuals with mental disorders can be complex as the patients' needs in three areas (biological, psychological and social) have to be assessed and met. Usually, all complex cases are assigned a care coordinator and managed under a care programme approach (CPA) process. These terms are explained below.

- Care coordinator:
  - they can be any member of the team;
  - they should meet with their clients regularly;
  - their role is to coordinate the care of their patients by liaising with the various professionals involved in the care of these patients;
  - care coordinators lead on CPA meetings;
  - they are also responsible for the patients' care plans.
- Care programme approach:
  - the CPA process has four main aspects:
    - assessment – systematic arrangements for assessing the health and social needs of patients under secondary psychiatric care,
    - a care plan – the formation of a care plan to address all identified health and social care needs,
    - a key worker (or care coordinator) to keep in touch with the patient and monitor their care,
    - regular reviews to check on progress and agree any changes to the care plan.
- CPA review meetings:
  - these are meetings that take place at least 6-monthly;
  - they involve all members of the multidisciplinary team;
  - the patient is the focus of these meetings;
  - patients' families/carers are invited to attend CPA meetings.

At CPA meetings, the management of the patient (both pharmacological and non-pharmacological), progress, risks and a crisis plan in case of a relapse are discussed. Longer-term management plans are put in place and further review dates agreed.

Mental health assessment and service provision

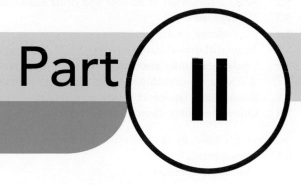

Part II

Mental health disorders

4. Organic mental disorders 33

4.1 Delirium 33
4.2 Dementia 38
4.3 Pseudodementia 42
4.4 Alzheimer's disease 42
4.5 Vascular dementia 45
4.6 Mixed dementia 47
4.7 Lewy body dementia 47
4.8 Dementia in Pick's disease (a frontotemporal dementia) 48
4.9 Old age psychiatry 49
4.10 Late-onset schizophrenia 49
4.11 Late-onset bipolar disorder 50
4.12 Late-onset depressive disorder 51
4.13 Suicide in older people 52
4.14 Substance misuse among older adults 53
4.15 Organic dementia 53
4.16 Head injury 55
4.17 Damage to specific areas of the brain 56
4.18 Endocrine disorders 56
4.19 Metabolic disorders 58
4.20 Nutritional disorders 59
4.21 Autoimmune disorders 60

5. Substance misuse   62
5.1   Assessment of substance misuse   62
5.2   Acute intoxication of alcohol and other substances   64
5.3   Harmful use   66
5.4   Dependence syndrome   67
5.5   Acute withdrawal state   70
5.6   Psychotic disorder associated with substance misuse   70
5.7   Wernicke's encephalopathy and Korsakoff's syndrome   71
5.8   Residual and late-onset psychotic disorder   73
5.9   Other commonly abused substances   74

6. Schizophrenia and delusional disorders   77
6.1   Schizophrenia   77
6.2   Delusional disorders   89
6.3   Acute and transient psychotic disorders   93
6.4   Induced delusional disorder (folie à deux)   96
6.5   Schizoaffective disorders   97

7. Affective disorders   100
7.1   Manic episode   100
7.2   Depressive episode   104
7.3   Recurrent depressive disorder   113
7.4   Bipolar affective disorder   115
7.5   Other affective disorders   119

8. Anxiety and neuroses   123
8.1   Generalized anxiety disorder   123
8.2   Mixed anxiety and depression   125
8.3   Panic disorder   126
8.4   Specific phobia   128
8.5   Agoraphobia   129
8.6   Social phobia   130
8.7   Obsessive–compulsive disorder   132
8.8   Acute stress reaction   134
8.9   Post-traumatic stress disorder   135
8.10   Adjustment disorder   137
8.11   Somatization disorder   138
8.12   Hypochondriacal disorder   139
8.13   Somatoform autonomic dysfunction   140
8.14   Somatoform pain disorder   140

9. Behavioural syndromes associated with
   physiological disturbance   142
   9.1   Eating disorders   142
   9.2   Sleep disorders   147
   9.3   Psychosexual disorders   151
   9.4   Disorders related to the puerperium and menstruation 155

10. Disorders of adult personality   162
   10.1   Definition   162
   10.2   Epidemiology   162
   10.3   Aetiology   162
   10.4   Classification   163
   10.5   Treatment   168
   10.6   Prognosis   169

11. Learning disability and child and adolescent
    disorders   170
   11.1   General learning disability   170
   11.2   Down's syndrome   174
   11.3   Fragile X syndrome   175
   11.4   Fetal alcohol syndrome   175
   11.5   Psychiatric assessment in children   176
   11.6   Conduct disorders   176
   11.7   Oppositional defiant disorder   178
   11.8   Disorders of social functioning   178
   11.9   Hyperkinetic disorder   179
   11.10 Autism   181
   11.11 Asperger's syndrome   182
   11.12 Tourette's syndrome   183
   11.13 Non-organic enuresis   184
   11.14 Adolescent depression   185
   11.15 Adolescent suicide and deliberate self-harm   186
   11.16 Adolescent substance misuse   187

12. Forensic psychiatry   189
   12.1   Assessment   189
   12.2   Crime and mental health   189
   12.3   Legal competence   191

13. Pharmacotherapy   192
   13.1   Antidepressants   192
   13.2   Antipsychotics   197
   13.3   Mood stabilizers   206
   13.4   Anxiolytics and hypnotics   209

14. Electroconvulsive therapy and psychotherapy   213
14.1   Electroconvulsive therapy   213
14.2   Psychotherapy   215

15. Psychiatric emergencies   218
15.1   Suicide   218
15.2   Self-harm   221
15.3   Lithium toxicity   223
15.4   Neuroleptic malignant syndrome   224
15.5   Acute dystonic reaction   227
15.6   Acute alcohol withdrawal state with delirium   228
15.7   Aggression and agitation   231

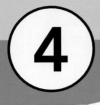

Organic mental disorders

4.1 DELIRIUM

> **MICRO-case**
> A 79-year-old woman is admitted following a fall. She lives alone and is believed to have been lying in her bedroom for 3 days. She has a suspected fracture of the right neck of femur. When assessed by the Foundation Doctor she appears confused and does not remember what has happened. She becomes agitated as she is asked more questions and tries to hit the nurse who is doing her observations. On examination she is dehydrated and seems underweight. Her right leg is shorter than her left and is externally rotated. The patient screams in pain if anyone tries to move it. When the patient's daughter arrives an hour later she says her mother is 'not normally confused and is fully independent'. When the patient sees her daughter she becomes less agitated and seems less confused. She allows a cannula to be put in so fluids and analgesia can be given and becomes more coherent as she is in less pain and becomes hydrated.
>
> **Learning points**
>
> - A collateral history is very important when a confused patient presents.
> - The importance of recognizing correctible causes of delirium, in this case pain and dehydration.

EPIDEMIOLOGY

- Prevalence in hospital:
    - medically ill patients: 10–30%;
    - elderly patients: 10–40%;
    - terminally ill patients: 80%.
- Higher prevalence the more elderly the population.
- About 33–66% of patients with delirium are unidentified.

AETIOLOGY

- Pathophysiology is poorly understood (see Fig. 4.1).

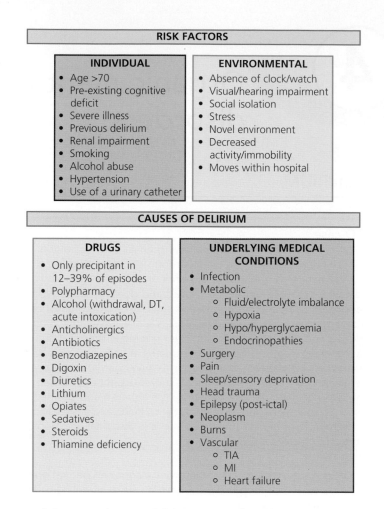

Fig. 4.1 Risk factors and causes of delirium. DT, delirium tremens; MI, myocardial infarction; TIA, transient ischaemic attack.

MICRO-print

There is evidence that neurotransmitter disturbances (acetylcholine deficiency and dopamine excess) may cause delirium. Reduced activity of plasma esterases in delirium have also been shown. These play an important role in drug metabolism, which may explain why many cases of delirium are caused by medication.

CLINICAL FEATURES

> **MICRO-facts**
>
> Core features of delirium:
> 1. Disturbance of consciousness.
> 2. Impairment in cognitive function.
> 3. Occurs over a short period (rapid onset, short duration).
> 4. Fluctuations in severity and presentation over the course of the day.

- Develops over hours or days.
- Fluctuating symptoms that are usually worse at night.
- Impaired cognitive function:
    - impairment in short-term memory with relatively intact long-term memory;
    - disorientation in time, place and person.
- Impaired consciousness:
    - decreased awareness of environment;
    - reduced attention.
- Disturbed perception:
    - illusions and visual hallucinations are common and may lead to aggression.
- Disturbance of sleep–wake cycle:
    - insomnia;
    - disturbing dreams and nightmares that may continue as hallucinations upon waking.
- Physical function:
    - unpredictable shifts from hypoactivity to hyperactivity;
    - increased reaction time;
    - incoherent speech.
- Disturbance of mood and affect:
    - ranges from apathy and anxiety to terror.
- Objective evidence of underlying systemic or cerebral disease that can be presumed to be responsible for clinical manifestations.
- Delirium may be hypoactive, hyperactive or mixed (Table 4.1).

CLINICAL ASSESSMENT

It is important to take a third-party history from, for example, a relative, carer or general practitioner (GP).
- Screening questions to include in history:
    - onset and course of confusion;
    - previous episodes to exclude pre-existing dementia;

Table 4.1 Features of hyperactive and hypoactive delirium.

	HYPERACTIVE	HYPOACTIVE
Cognition	Decreased	Decreased
Affect	Agitated	Withdrawn, apathetic
Motor activity	Increased, wandering and restless	Decreased, lethargic
Prognosis	Better	Poorer

- any psychotic thoughts (in delirium these are simple and fleeting, exclude schizophrenia where ideas are complex and persisting);
- previous intellectual function (i.e. ability to manage own affairs);
- comorbid illnesses;
- full drug history including recent drug cessation (see drugs in causes);
- bowel and urinary symptoms, including catheter use, to exclude constipation and infection;
- exclude systemic features of infection;
- activities of daily living including whether the patient normally has carers;
- pre-admission social circumstances;
- sensory deficits and aids used (e.g. glasses, hearing aids);
- alcohol history, exclude delirium tremens (see Chapter 15 Psychiatric emergencies, Acute alcohol withdrawal state with delirium).
- Assess cognitive function using a standardized test that can be repeated to look for improvement/deterioration, for example:
  - abbreviated mental test score (AMT, out of 10 points);
  - short confusion assessment method (CAM);
  - mini-mental state examination (MMSE).
- Differential diagnosis (Table 4.2).

Table 4.2 Differences between depression, dementia and delirium.

	DELIRIUM	DEMENTIA	DEPRESSION
Onset	Rapid	Gradual	Varied
Course	Fluctuating	Progressive	Diurnal variation
Consciousness	Impaired	Clear	Generally clear
Psychosis	Common	Common	May occur (in keeping with mood)
Memory and attention	Short-term memory affected and fluctuating attention	Poor memory and inattention	Short-term and working memory often impaired and poor attention

INVESTIGATIONS

- Bloods:
    - full blood count (FBC) and C-reactive protein (CRP): to determine if infection is causing delirium;
    - urea and electrolytes (U&E): to determine if renal impairment or electrolyte disturbances (e.g. hypercalcaemia, hyponatraemia) are causing delirium;
    - liver function tests (LFTs): to determine if liver failure or infection is causing delirium;
    - thyroid function tests (TFTs): to determine if thyroid dysfunction is causing delirium;
    - B_{12} and folate: important in patients with high alcohol intake and malnutrition;
    - glucose: to determine if hyperglycaemia or hypoglycaemia is causing delirium.
- Septic screen:
    - chest X-ray: to determine if pneumonia is causing delirium;
    - urinalysis: to determine if urinary tract infection (UTI) or renal dysfunction is causing delirium;
    - blood cultures: to determine if septicaemia is causing delirium;
    - specific tests as appropriate if not excluded by tests above:
        - sputum culture,
        - mid-stream urine (MSU) culture,
        - lumbar puncture (if signs of meningism).
- Other:
    - electrocardiogram (ECG): arrhythmias, bundle branch block, other abnormalities;
    - pulse oximetry: hypoxia;
    - arterial blood gases: lactate levels may show infection, pH and base excess may show acidosis/alkalosis;
    - computed tomography (CT):
        - if focal neurological symptoms exist,
        - after a fall,
        - if a head injury is suspected.

MANAGEMENT

- If possible correct the underlying cause.
- All medications should be reviewed on a daily basis and those not essential should be stopped.
- Environmental:
    - make sure patients have any aids needed (e.g. glasses, hearing aid);
    - allow clear orientation (e.g. clock, calendar, schedule, sign with named nurse);

- try to minimize sleep disturbance and ensure appropriate lighting for time of day;
- encourage early mobilization;
- ensure adequate diet and hydration and avoid catheterization.
- Pharmacological:
  - **only** if a patient is severely distressed, is a danger to themselves or others or needs essential treatment;
  - haloperidol is the recommended treatment for agitation:
    - 0.5 mg orally as initial dose, up to 5–10 mg in 24 hours,
    - can be given intramuscularly (IM),
    - doses above 3 mg can predispose patients to extrapyramidal symptoms so procyclidine 5 mg oral (po)/IM can be prescribed;
  - an alternative to haloperidol in patients with Parkinson's disease or Lewy body dementia is lorazepam 0.5–1 mg orally up to 3 mg in 24 hours.

PROGNOSIS

- Among hospital inpatients less than half will have recovered at the time of discharge and delirium can persist for many months afterwards.
- Communication with the family and GP about the condition and prognosis is important.
- Evidence shows a worse physical and mental recovery in the following year with more time spent in hospital or rehabilitation centres.
- Most patients will make a full recovery; however, memories of the period can be very disturbing for the patient.

CAPACITY

- Patients suffering from delirium should have their capacity to make specific decisions assessed and documented.
- A patient suffering from delirium is unlikely to have the capacity to make a decision regarding their treatment.
- If treatment is urgent or for a life-threatening condition then the treating team can provide the required treatment acting in the patient's best interest.

4.2 DEMENTIA

MICRO-case

A 78-year-old man is brought into the emergency department (ED) after being found wandering in the street in his dressing gown in the middle of winter. He tells you that he is fine but he just got a little lost on his way home. When you ask where he was going he is not sure but starts to tell

continued...

continued...

you about the shops that used to be near his house. He can tell you his name but the address he gives you is 20 years out of date. When you perform a MMSE he scores 11/30. His wife is found and comes to the ED. She tells you he has been forgetful for many years but has recently started wandering and trying to go to work even though he retired 15 years ago. He can still wash and dress himself but needs prompting to do so and it is no longer safe to let him cook as he has previously left the gas cooker on. She has not seen anyone about this as she thinks it is just part of growing old. She is worried because recently her husband has started getting angry when she tells him what he needs to do and has tried to hit her.

Learning point

- Families may need a lot of support if they are to continue caring for patients with dementia.

EPIDEMIOLOGY

- Male to female ratio: male < female (possibly because of a shorter male lifespan).
- Prevalence:
    - age 65–69 years: 1.5%;
    - age 70–74 years: 2.4%;
    - age 75–79 years: 6%;
    - age 80–84 years: 13.3%;
    - age 85–89 years: 20%.

AETIOLOGY

- Depends on the cause of dementia (see individual conditions).

MICRO-facts

Dementia is a progressive failure of many cerebral functions without clouding of consciousness. It may be accompanied or preceded by a deterioration in emotional control, social function and motivation.

CLINICAL FEATURES

- Cognitive impairment:
    - memory impairment (especially short-term);
    - calculations and problem-solving;
    - judgement, attention and orientation;
    - language.
- Decline in self-care and ability to perform activities of daily living (ADLs).

Mental health disorders

- Psychiatric and behavioural changes:
  - depression;
  - hallucinations and delusions;
  - personality change;
  - emotional change;
  - social withdrawal.

HISTORY AND SCREENING

- Take a history from the patient and also family/main carer.
- Onset:
  - if sudden assess for delirium.
- Course:
  - if short course think of depression as dementia is irreversible.
- Ability to perform activities of daily living.
- Medical history:
  - vascular risk factors;
  - family history.
- Drug history:
  - are they compliant with medication?
  - are they at risk of overdose by duplicating doses?
  - could any medications impair cognition?
- Support network.
- Screening for depression (pseudodementia) **must** be performed (see later under Pseudodementia and Chapter 7 Affective disorders, Depressive episode).
- Screen for dementia using a tool such as the MMSE:
  - scores out of 30:
    - normal ageing = 27–30,
    - mild impairment = 24–26,
    - early dementia = 21–23,
    - moderate dementia = 10–20,
    - severe dementia = below 10;
  - important to remember that the score may not be accurate for patients whose first language is not English and for those who have a physical disability and/or sensory impairments.

MICRO-print

Other tools used in dementia:

- Clinical dementia rating – global assessment;
- Neuropsychiatric inventory – behavioural and psychological assessment;
- Bristol scale – ADLs.

INVESTIGATIONS

- Baseline investigations to be performed to exclude organic causes:
  - FBC to exclude infection and anaemia;
  - U&E to exclude uraemia and electrolyte imbalance;
  - glucose to exclude hypoglycaemia or diabetes mellitus;
  - calcium to exclude hypercalcaemia;
  - LFTs to exclude liver failure;
  - TFTs to exclude thyroid dysfunction;
  - serum B_{12} and folate (important as deficiencies may cause confusion);
  - syphilis screen to exclude neurosyphilis (if suspected);
  - human immunodeficiency virus (HIV) screen to exclude HIV/acquired immune deficiency syndrome (AIDS) (if suspected).
- Exclude delirium if onset is sudden (see section on Delirium above).
- CT or magnetic resonance imaging (MRI) scan: to exclude focal pathology and diagnose subtype of dementia (see individual subtypes).

MANAGEMENT

- Specific management is based on the subtype of dementia (see below).
- Patients should be referred to a specialist memory clinic and other relevant services for management (e.g. occupational therapy and social services).
- Discuss diagnosis and implications with patient, family and carers.
- Management is initially non-pharmacological; drugs are used when these measures have failed.
- Risperidone (an atypical antipsychotic) is licensed in the UK for short-term treatment of persistent aggression in Alzheimer's disease.
- The use of antipsychotics in dementia is associated with increased mortality, hastening of cognitive decline and an increased risk of stroke.
- Benzodiazepine use is associated with worsening cognitive decline, falls and hip fractures.

PROGNOSIS

- Dementia is a chronic and progressive disease with no cure.
- It is important to consider issues surrounding future capacity and make sure these are addressed with the family.

CAPACITY

- While a person still has capacity it is important to discuss with them the options for future decisions:
  - advance statements for certain situations;
  - advance decisions to refuse treatment;
  - lasting power of attorney.

Mental health disorders

4.3 PSEUDODEMENTIA

- Symptoms and signs of dementia present but no damage to the brain.
- Caused by **severe depression** which can be treated with **antidepressants**.
- How to differentiate: Table 4.3

Table 4.3 Differences between dementia and pseudodementia.

	PSEUDODEMENTIA	DEMENTIA
Onset	Quick	Slow
Mood	Depressed	Normal
Weight	Weight loss owing to loss of appetite	May decrease with self-neglect
Daytime variation	Diurnal variation in mood	Behaviour is worse and motor activity increases in the evening (sundowning in Alzheimer's)
Recall	May recall when prompted	No recall if prompted
Treatment	Recovery with antidepressants	No change with antidepressants
Insight	Good	Little or none

4.4 ALZHEIMER'S DISEASE

EPIDEMIOLOGY

- 50–60% of dementia sufferers.
- Male to female ratio: male < female (possibly because of a shorter male lifespan).
- Prevalence:
    - age 40–64 years: 1 in 1400;
    - age 65–69 years: 1 in 100;
    - age 70–79 years: 1 in 25;
    - age 80+ years: 1 in 6.
- There is a 3.5 times higher risk of developing Alzheimer's disease if one first-degree relative affected.

AETIOLOGY

- Genetic factors:
    - early-onset Alzheimer's (before age 60 years) can be associated with three genes:

- genetic fault in *amyloid precursor protein (APP)* gene on chromosome 21 leads to build-up of amyloid in the brain (very rare),
    - genetic fault in one of the presenilin genes, *PS-1* on chromosome 14 and *PS-2* on chromosome 1 (very rare, occurs in familial early-onset disease);
  - in late-onset Alzheimer's the gene for apolipoprotein E (ApoE) on chromosome 19 is important:
    - ApoE4 is associated with an increased risk,
    - ApoE2 appears to have a protective effect.
- Neuroanatomical abnormalities:
  - findings on CT imaging:
    - shrinkage of cerebral hemispheres,
    - widened sulci,
    - enlarged ventricles;
  - neuronal damage:
    - senile plaques made of beta-amyloid and degenerating nerve endings,
    - neurofibrillary tangles,
    - loss of enzymes which help make certain neurotransmitters, especially acetylcholine.
- Dietary theories (these are still being researched):
  - vitamin B_{12} and folate:
    - low levels of dietary folate and B_{12} cause high levels of homocysteine in the blood, which has been linked with memory loss;
  - omega-3 fatty acids:
    - those who eat one to two portions of oily fish a week found to have lower levels of Alzheimer's disease than those who eat none;
  - anti-oxidants (vitamins C and E):
    - both are anti-oxidants which clear free radicals,
    - some evidence to show those with a high intake from natural sources have a lower level of dementia.
- Dementia in Down's syndrome:
  - by the age of 40 years almost all people with Down's syndrome have some signs of Alzheimer's disease as they have an extra copy of the *APP* gene on chromosome 21.

CLINICAL FEATURES

- Initial memory lapses with difficulty using language.
- Deterioration in ability to plan, organize and complete household tasks and ADLs.
- Mood swings and gradual withdrawal from social interaction.

- Inability to recognize friends and family and loss of short-term memory.
- Gradual progression (if sudden deterioration consider vascular dementia).

HISTORY AND SCREENING

See section on Dementia for general questions.

- Onset: patient and family are usually unable to say exactly when memory problems began.
- Course: gradual and progressive.
- Mood: aggression is common, especially towards those providing care.
- Language: difficulties with word finding, fluency and increasing circum-stantiality.
- Motor function: in severe disease may have problems with continence, eating and frontal reflexes may reappear.

INVESTIGATIONS

See section on Dementia for general questions.

- MMSE (limited by lack of frontal lobe assessment).
- Addenbrooke's cognitive examination (incorporates MMSE and frontal lobe assessment).
- CT scan should show neuroanatomical abnormalities as described above (Fig. 4.2).

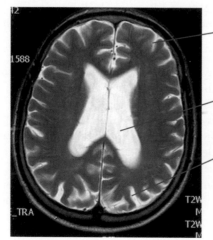

Frontal lobes sulci relatively spared

Ventriculomegaly secondary to brain atrophy

Dilated sulci of parietal lobes indicating posterior cortical atrophy

Fig. 4.2 T2-weighted MRI scan showing features of Alzheimer's disease.

MANAGEMENT

For non-pharmacological management see section on Dementia.
- Pharmacological therapy:
  - used when MMSE score is between 26 and 12;
  - use acetylcholinesterase inhibitors which:
    - stabilize condition initially,
    - delay decline,
    - postpone onset of severe dementia;
  - examples: donepezil (once daily), galantamine (twice daily), rivastigmine (twice daily; available in oral tablets and patch);
  - common side-effects:
    - excessive cholinergic effects such as nausea, diarrhoea, dizziness, urinary incontinence and insomnia,
    - other side-effects include headache, parasympathetic stimulation and cardiac adverse events;
  - when MMSE score is less than 12:
    - memantine is indicated for moderately severe to severe dementia,
    - memantine is a N-methyl-D-aspartate (NMDA) receptor antagonist and has neuroprotective properties,
    - not curative.

PROGNOSIS

- Gradual decline in memory, cognitive and motor function.
- Life expectancy not shortened.
- Acetylcholinesterase inhibitors slow decline; however, once the drugs stop working function may deteriorate rapidly over months.

4.5 VASCULAR DEMENTIA

EPIDEMIOLOGY

- 20–30% of dementia sufferers.
- Usually occurs in people with other vascular disease.
- Prevalence:
  - age 65–69 years: 0.3%;
  - age 70–74 years: 0.7%;
  - age 75–79 years: 1.4%;
  - age 80–84 years: 2.4%;
  - age 85+ years: 3.6%;

AETIOLOGY

- Neuropathological abnormalities:

- previously known as 'multi-infarct dementia' as it can be caused by emboli, leading to cerebral infarcts;
  - small-vessel atherosclerosis.
- Risk factors:
  - diet high in cholesterol;
  - smoking;
  - obesity;
  - hypertension;
  - diabetes mellitus.

CLINICAL FEATURES

- Patients can experience sudden decline and then a plateau.
- Emboli can cause sudden decline with subsequent small improvements in specific areas, for example loss of speech with improvement over time.
- Uneven decline in functions, for example severe memory loss but language relatively intact.
- See section on Dementia.

HISTORY AND SCREENING

- See section on Dementia for general questions.
- Onset: can be sudden because of a vascular event.
- Course: stepped, with sudden decline.
- Physical history: history of hypertension, coronary artery disease, stroke, peripheral vascular disease and diabetes mellitus.
- Drug history: is the patient on preventative medication to modify risk factors?

INVESTIGATIONS

- Baseline investigations as in dementia (see section on Dementia).
- ECG: if atrial fibrillation (AF), consider anticoagulation.
- Carotid Doppler: to assess for stenosis; if present carotid endarterectomy may help prevent future events.
- Check cholesterol, lipid and screen for diabetes mellitus.
- Measure blood pressure to assess for uncontrolled hypertension.
- CT scan: lacunar and multiple infarcts visible (Fig. 4.3).

MANAGEMENT

- Modify risk factor profile if possible:
  - control hypertension;
  - statin if low-density lipoprotein (LDL) cholesterol raised;
  - tighten glucose control if diabetic.

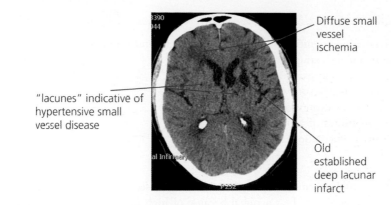

Diffuse small vessel ischemia

"lacunes" indicative of hypertensive small vessel disease

Old established deep lacunar infarct

Fig. 4.3 Computed tomography (CT) scan showing features of vascular dementia.

- For general management see section on Dementia.

PROGNOSIS

- Progressive dementia with no cure.

4.6 MIXED DEMENTIA

- It is possible to have a mixture of Alzheimer's type dementia and vascular dementia.
- Specialist advice on best management is needed.

4.7 LEWY BODY DEMENTIA

EPIDEMIOLOGY

- Comprises 15–20% of all dementia cases.
- Male to female ratio: 1:1.

AETIOLOGY

- Neuropathological abnormalities:
  - widespread Lewy bodies present (abnormal aggregates of protein that develop inside neurons present in the cerebral cortex);
  - Lewy bodies also occur in Parkinson's disease but are mostly limited to the substantia nigra.

Mental health disorders

CLINICAL FEATURES

- Fluctuating cognitive impairment over weeks and months.
- Spontaneous extrapyramidal symptoms:
  - shuffling gait;
  - reduced arm swing;
  - blank expression;
  - stiffness of walking.
- Visual hallucinations.

MANAGEMENT

- No specific treatment – for general treatment see section on Dementia.
- Antipsychotics are best avoided because of high incidence of neuroleptic sensitivity syndrome.

4.8 DEMENTIA IN PICK'S DISEASE (A FRONTOTEMPORAL DEMENTIA)

EPIDEMIOLOGY

- Male to female ratio: male < female (slight difference).
- Peak age of onset at 50–60 years.

AETIOLOGY

- Neuropathological abnormalities:
  - progressive destruction of neurons with accumulation of protein-forming Pick bodies;
  - selective atrophy of frontal and temporal lobe with knife-blade atrophy of the gyri.

MICRO-facts

Diagnostic criteria (ICD-10):

- Must have general symptoms of dementia.
- Slow onset and steady deterioration.
- Predominance of frontal lobe involvement:
  - emotional blunting;
  - coarsening of social behaviour;
  - disinhibition;
  - apathy or restlessness;
  - aphasia.
- In early stages memory relatively intact.

CLINICAL FEATURES

- Differential diagnosis:
  - Alzheimer's dementia:
    - in Pick's disease, character and behaviour changes develop before signs of memory loss.

DIAGNOSIS

- Can only be diagnosed by autopsy.

4.9 OLD AGE PSYCHIATRY

Mental illness is common in the older adult population. The most frequently encountered conditions are delirium, depression and dementia. However, other major disorders such as schizophrenia, bipolar affective disorder and substance misuse do still occur.

4.10 LATE-ONSET SCHIZOPHRENIA

DEFINITION

- Late onset schizophrenia: 40–59 years.
- Very late onset schizophrenia: over 60 years.

EPIDEMIOLOGY

- Prevalence: < 1%.
- Male to female ratio: male < female.

AETIOLOGY

- Sensory impairment (e.g. deafness).
- Social isolation.
- Paranoid or schizoid personality.

CLINICAL FEATURES

- Onset is usually insidious.
- In 20% of cases, only delusions are seen.
- First-rank symptoms are less common when compared with younger adults.
- Common delusion themes: persecutory and misidentification.
- Auditory hallucination in 75% of cases.
- Visual hallucinations in some patients.
- Early cognitive impairment in some patients.

Mental health disorders

INVESTIGATIONS

- Larger ventricles on CT brain scan.

DIFFERENTIAL DIAGNOSIS

- Delusional disorder.
- Dementia.
- Delirium.

MANAGEMENT

- The use of antipsychotics is associated with an increased risk of cerebro-vascular accident.
- First-generation antipsychotics are also associated with increased extrapyramidal side-effects.
- Patients should be provided with adequate information on the risk and benefits of antipsychotics and empowered to make an informed decision.

PROGNOSIS

- Response to antipsychotics is usually good, although careful monitoring is required for side-effects.

4.11 LATE-ONSET BIPOLAR DISORDER

EPIDEMIOLOGY

- Prevalence: 0.1% in over 65-year-olds.
- Male to female ratio: 1:2.

AETIOLOGY

- More common for depression to switch to mania in older people.
- Cerebral insult is a common cause.

CLINICAL FEATURES

- Less flight of ideas and hyperactivity when compared with adults with bipolar disorder.
- More irritable and with paranoid delusions.

MANAGEMENT

- A second-generation antipsychotic (e.g. risperidone, olanzapine) is considered as the first-line agent.
- Consider lithium as a second-line agent.
- Maintenance level of lithium for elderly is around 0.4–0.6 mmol/L.

4.12 LATE-ONSET DEPRESSIVE DISORDER

EPIDEMIOLOGY

- Prevalence:
    - in the community: 3%;
    - GP clinic: 30%;
    - residential care: 40%;
    - medical ward: 45%.
- Male to female ratio: 1:2 (mild depression), 1:1 (severe depression).

AETIOLOGY

- Cancer.
- Cardiovascular diseases.
- Central nervous system disorder.
- Living alone or unmarried.
- Widowhood, especially after first year of death of the spouse.
- Presence of dementia.

CLINICAL FEATURES

- Psychomotor retardation or agitation.
- Depressive delusions (e.g. poverty and nihilistic).
- Derogatory and obscene auditory hallucinations.
- Nervousness and irritability.
- Cognitive impairment is common (70% of elderly with depression).

INVESTIGATIONS

- Geriatric depression scale (GDS).
- MRI:
    - deep white matter changes;
    - enlargement of ventricles.

MANAGEMENT

- Psychological therapy:
    - psychotherapy can be very effective.
- Pharmacological therapy:
    - antidepressants:
        - selective serotonin re-uptake inhibitors (SSRIs) are better tolerated than tricyclic antidepressants (TCAs);
        - SSRIs increase the risk of gastrointestinal bleeding, particularly in elderly patients taking non-steroidal anti-inflammatory drugs (NSAIDs) or warfarin;

Mental health disorders

    – elderly patients are prone to develop hyponatraemia;
    – poorer treatment response and take longer to respond
       (6–8 weeks).

- Other therapies:
  - electroconvulsive therapy (ECT) is effective in 80% of severe depression, especially for those with anxiety and agitation (it should be noted that the presence of a cardiac pacemaker is **not** an absolute contraindication).

PROGNOSIS

- Organic brain disorder and chronic depression may lead to poor prognosis.
- Long-term prognosis is unfavourable for 40% of cases.

4.13 SUICIDE IN OLDER PEOPLE

EPIDEMIOLOGY

- 25% of suicides are committed by the elderly.
- Parasuicide (deliberate self-harm) is rare among the elderly.

RISK FACTORS

- Male gender.
- Cancer.
- Cerebrovascular accidents.
- Epilepsy.
- Multiple sclerosis.
- Social isolation.

CLINICAL FEATURES

- Common methods include hanging, drowning and overdose.
- Suicide among older people may take place within the first few hours of admission and within weeks after discharge.
- Less common in those staying in residential care.

MANAGEMENT

- Management of attempted suicide and deliberate self-harm in the elderly should be taken as evidence of suicidal intent until proven otherwise.
- Old-age psychiatrists or geriatricians need to treat underlying cause such as depressive disorder or medical problems.

4.14 SUBSTANCE MISUSE AMONG OLDER ADULTS

EPIDEMIOLOGY

- Male to female ratio: 2–6:1.
- Men start drinking in adulthood and continue into old age.
- Female gender is a risk factor for late-onset alcohol misuse.

AETIOLOGY

- Precipitated by sudden access to excess time and money after retirement.
- Higher social class is a risk factor for late-onset alcohol misuse.
- The presence of depression and anxiety are also risk factors.
- Associated with cognitive impairment.
- See Chapter 5 Substance misuse for further information.

4.15 ORGANIC DEMENTIA

CREUTZFELDT–JAKOB DISEASE

- Aetiology:
  - prion disease:
    - induces abnormal folding of prion proteins in the central nervous system,
    - leads to gliosis, synaptic and neuronal loss;
  - can be transmissible person to person.
- Clinical features:
  - symptoms:
    - early signs: mood changes, memory loss and apathy,
    - progressing to severe dementia,
    - slow and slurred speech, clumsiness and loss of balance,
    - loss of all abilities and function needing full-time care;
  - different forms of Creutzfeldt–Jakob disease (CJD) are shown in Table 4.4.
- Prognosis:
  - very poor prognosis as there is no treatment.

DEMENTIA WITH HIV AND AIDS

- Epidemiology:
  - depends on how well suppressed HIV is with anti-retrovirals;
  - may occur in up to 40% of patients.

Table 4.4 Different forms of Creutzfeldt–Jakob disease (CJD).

	SPORADIC (CLASSICAL)	FAMILIAL	VARIANT
Age at presentation	Mainly over 50s	From 20 years of age	Young age
Cause	Not known	Genetic – autosomal dominant inheritance	Caused by prion infection from other animals
Progression	Rapidly progressing dementia	Longer course, 2–10 years	Length of illness tends to be around 14 months

- Clinical features:
  - cognitive – poor concentration and memory loss affecting social function;
  - motor – initially poor balance, clumsiness and incoordination;
  - advanced – hyper-reflexia, leg weakness, seizures and incontinence;
  - behaviour – personality changes.
- Management:
  - highly active anti-retroviral therapy (HAART) may halt the changes and can sometimes reverse cognitive impairment.

MICRO-facts

- Emotional lability with agitation, disinhibition and hyperactivity can occur.
- Symptoms must be distinguished from primary mood disorders.

NEUROSYPHILIS

- Aetiology:
  - occurs after 10–20 years of untreated syphilis infection;
  - caused by the bacteria *Treponema pallidum*.
- Clinical features (include):
  - dementia;
  - confusion;
  - irritability;
  - poor concentration.
- Management:
  - intravenous benzylpenicillin sodium (seek specialist advice).

VIRAL ENCEPHALITIS

- Aetiology:
  - psychiatric symptoms arising during an episode of viral encephalitis and persisting after treatment of the infection is complete;
  - commonly herpes simplex infection.
- Clinical features:
  - personality change;
  - dementia;
  - anxiety;
  - depression;
  - in children, behavioural disorders may occur.

4.16 HEAD INJURY

SHORT-TERM EFFECTS

- Clinical features:
  - impairment of consciousness;
  - amnesia:
    - retrograde (from before injury),
    - anterograde (increased length of amnesia after injury is consistent with increased severity of injury);
  - post-injury psychosis or disturbed behaviour.

LONG-TERM EFFECTS

- Clinical features:
  - personality change related to area of brain affected (see section on Damage to specific areas of the brain below);
  - cognitive impairment;
  - epilepsy;
  - mood, anxiety or psychotic disorders.

PUNCH DRUNK SYNDROME

- Aetiology:
  - follows repeated blows to the head (e.g. in boxers);
  - cerebral atrophy is common.
- Clinical features:
  - dementia;
  - change in personality with increased irritability;
  - movement disorder consistent with cerebellar dysfunction.

4.17 DAMAGE TO SPECIFIC AREAS OF THE BRAIN

AETIOLOGY

- Psychiatric symptoms may arise because of pathology in a specific area of the brain:
    - primary or metastatic tumours;
    - cerebrovascular disease (stroke);
    - cerebral abscess.

CLINICAL FEATURES

Clinical features are outlined in Fig. 4.4.

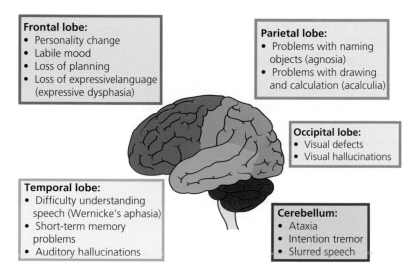

Frontal lobe:
- Personality change
- Labile mood
- Loss of planning
- Loss of expressivelanguage (expressive dysphasia)

Parietal lobe:
- Problems with naming objects (agnosia)
- Problems with drawing and calculation (acalculia)

Occipital lobe:
- Visual defects
- Visual hallucinations

Temporal lobe:
- Difficulty understanding speech (Wernicke's aphasia)
- Short-term memory problems
- Auditory hallucinations

Cerebellum:
- Ataxia
- Intention tremor
- Slurred speech

Fig. 4.4 Clinical features of damage to different areas of the brain.

4.18 ENDOCRINE DISORDERS

Common endocrine conditions which lead to psychiatric symptoms are outlined in Table 4.5.

Table 4.5 Common endocrine conditions that present with psychiatric symptoms.

CONDITION	PSYCHIATRIC SYMPTOMS	OTHER SYMPTOMS	CAUSE	TEST
Hyperthyroidism	Anxiety, irritability, behaviour change	Heat intolerance, tremor, weight loss, palpitations	High thyroxine, low TSH (normally)	Thyroid function tests
Hypothyroidism	Depression, malaise, poor libido, psychosis	Cold intolerance, weight gain, goitre, tiredness	Low thyroxine, high TSH (normally)	Thyroid function tests
Phaeochromocytoma	Anxiety or panic attacks	High blood pressure, sweating, tachycardia	Catecholamine excess	Measurement of urinary catecholamines and metabolites
Cushing's disease	Depression, insomnia, poor libido, psychosis	Bruising, central weight gain, striae, hirsutism	Glucocorticoid excess	24-hour urinary free cortisol test
Addison's disease	Depression, anorexia, malaise	Weight loss, pigmentation, wasting	Decreased glucocorticoids	Short ACTH stimulation test

ACTH, adrenocorticotropic hormone; TSH, thyroid-stimulating hormone.

Mental health disorders

4.19 METABOLIC DISORDERS

HYPOCALCAEMIA

- Aetiology:
  - vitamin D deficiency;
  - hypoparathyroidism;
  - acute pancreatitis;
  - alkalosis.

> **MICRO-facts**
>
> - Signs of hypocalcaemia:
>   - Chvostek's sign (unilateral twitching of face from tapping ear lobe);
>   - Trousseau's sign (spasm of the hand from inflated blood pressure cuff).

- Clinical features:
  - calcium < 2.12 mmol/L;
  - symptoms:
    - depression,
    - bone fractures,
    - twitching muscles,
    - arrhythmias;
  - ECG changes (prolonged QT and arrhythmias).
- Management:
  - vitamin D and calcium replacement.

HYPERCALCAEMIA

- Aetiology:
  - hyperparathyroidism;
  - malignancy;
  - excess vitamin D supplements;
  - sarcoidosis.

> **MICRO-facts**
>
> - Symptoms of hypercalcaemia:
>   - bones – bone pain/fractures;
>   - stones – renal calculi;
>   - moans – depression.

- Clinical features:
  - calcium >2.65 mmol/L;
  - ECG changes (short QT and arrhythmias).
- Management:
  - 0.9% saline continuously for 4–5 days;
  - rate dependent on level of dehydration and if heart/renal failure is present.

WILSON'S DISEASE

- Epidemiology:
  - incidence rate 3.3 per 100000.
- Aetiology:
  - a defective *APT7B* gene on chromosome 13 results in impaired copper transport and an accumulation of copper in the brain, liver and other organs;
  - autosomal recessive inheritance;
  - carrier frequency 1 in 90.
- Clinical features:
  - neuropsychiatric:
    - asymmetrical tremor,
    - schizophrenic and behavioural symptoms;
  - hepatic:
    - chronic active hepatitis leading to fulminant liver disease;
  - ophthalmic:
    - Kayser–Fleischer ring (copper deposited in the cornea) may be visible on slit lamp examination.
- Investigations:
  - 24-hour urinary copper excretion is increased;
  - liver biopsy: copper deposits;
  - genetic test is positive;
  - ceruloplasmin levels (serum carrier protein for copper) decreased.
- Management:
  - lifelong D-penicillamine.
- Prognosis:
  - neurological disease has only a limited reversibility with treatment.

4.20 NUTRITIONAL DISORDERS

VITAMIN B$_{12}$ DEFICIENCY

- Aetiology:
  - autoimmune in pernicious anaemia;
  - malabsorption (e.g. owing to Crohn's disease);
  - non-supplemented vegan diet (non-animal sources of B$_{12}$ are difficult to access).

Mental health disorders

- Clinical features:
  - irritability;
  - confusion;
  - psychosis;
  - dementia;
  - intellectual impairment.
- Management:
  - intramuscular hydroxocobalamin (as directed by a specialist, depending on severity).

AMNESIC SYNDROME

- Also known as Korsakoff's syndrome, Korsakoff's dementia and Korsakoff's psychosis (see Chapter 5 Substance misuse, Wernicke's encephalopathy and Korsakoff's syndrome).

4.21 AUTOIMMUNE DISORDERS

MULTIPLE SCLEROSIS

- Aetiology:
  - demyelination of the central nervous system.
- Clinical features:
  - non-psychiatric features include:
    - optic neuritis,
    - vertigo,
    - sensory deficits,
    - neurogenic bladder dysfunction;
  - depression is very common;
  - transient psychosis may occur;
  - early stage – cognitive impairment;
  - late stage – progressive dementia.

SYSTEMIC LUPUS ERYTHEMATOSUS

- Aetiology:
  - systemic lupus erythematosus (SLE) is a connective tissue disorder which may present with cerebral involvement.
- Clinical features:
  - delirium may occur;
  - depressive psychosis;
  - symptoms aggravated by steroid treatment.

SARCOIDOSIS

- Aetiology:
    - granulomas form in organs;
    - unknown aetiology;
    - around 5% of patients have involvement of the central nervous system.
- Clinical features:
    - cognitive decline;
    - depression;
    - psychosis.

Substance misuse

5.1 ASSESSMENT OF SUBSTANCE MISUSE

ALCOHOL HISTORY

- CAGE screening questions – (see Chapter 1 History and mental state examination, Psychiatric history).
- Determine the patient's drinking pattern:
    - What alcohol is drunk? (e.g. beer, cider, wine, etc.);
    - How much is drunk in units? (daily/weekly depending on drinking pattern);
    - Do they drink daily?
    - Where do they drink (home, pub)?
    - Do they drink alone or with others?
    - What time of day do they have their first drink?
    - Do they drink steadily or sometimes binge drink?

MICRO-facts

How to calculate alcohol units:

Units = [Strength (ABV) × Volume (mL)]/1000

e.g. pint of beer at 5.2% ABV: $5.2 \times 568/1000 = 2.95$

- Ask about features of alcohol dependence:
    - problems controlling alcohol intake – do you ever have just one drink?
    - primacy – is drinking important to you?
    - compulsion – do you feel an urge to drink?
    - tolerance – does alcohol have less of an effect on you now than it used to?
    - withdrawal – do you ever feel anxious or shaky when you have not had a drink? ('eye-openers' in the morning)?
    - persistent use despite evidence of harm (e.g. in individuals who have liver problems or mood problems) – are you intending on cutting down on your drinking?

Dependence syndrome is diagnosed only if three or more of the above features have been present together at some time in the previous year.

- Ask about the impact alcohol has had on the patient's life:
  - physical:
    - liver disease (e.g. cirrhosis, malignancy),
    - peripheral neuropathy;
  - mental:
    - depression,
    - cognitive difficulties,
    - encephalopathy;
  - social:
    - unemployment,
    - relationship breakdown (e.g. divorce),
    - debt problems;
  - legal:
    - drink driving,
    - drunk and disorderly behaviour.

DRUG HISTORY

- Determine the patient's drug-taking pattern:
  - what drugs are being taken?
  - how frequently are they taking drugs?
  - what volume of drugs is being taken?
  - how long have they been using at the current level?
  - how much money is being spent on drugs?
  - what effect do they want from the drug?
  - how the drugs are administered (are they injecting)?
- Features of opiate dependence:
  - the same features as alcohol dependence, but some specific symptoms are:
    - flu-like symptoms,
    - sweating.
- Ask about the impact drugs have had on the patient's life:
  - physical:
    - local infections, abscesses,
    - deep vein thrombosis,
    - bacterial endocarditis,
    - systemic infections, e.g. human immunodeficiency virus (HIV), hepatitis C;
  - mental:
    - psychosis,
    - anxiety;

Mental health disorders

- social:
  - debt problems,
  - relationship problems, e.g. divorce,
  - unemployment,
  - homelessness;
- legal:
  - drug offences,
  - theft,
  - prostitution.

5.2 ACUTE INTOXICATION OF ALCOHOL AND OTHER SUBSTANCES

DEFINITION

The ICD-10 definition is:

'A transient condition following the administration of alcohol or other psychoactive substance, resulting in disturbances in level of consciousness, cognition, perception, affect or behaviour, or other psychophysiological functions and responses.'

> **MICRO-reference**
> http://www.who.int/substance_abuse/terminology/ICD10Clinical-Diagnosis.pdf

EPIDEMIOLOGY

- More than 100000 people every year attend emergency departments with alcohol-related problems in the UK.

> **MICRO-reference**
> http://www.dh.gov.uk

RISK FACTORS

- Genetic factors.
- Male gender.
- Family history.
- Culture.
- Availability of the substance.
- Peer pressure.
- Deprivation.

CLINICAL FEATURES

- Altered conscious level, convulsions.
- Smell of alcohol, incoordination, aggression, agitation.
- Slurred speech.
- Labile mood – may be excessively happy or sad.
- Variable thoughts depending on the substance.
- Possible perceptual distortions – hallucinations likely if hallucinogenic substances used.
- Slowed, impaired judgment.
- Insight may be poor.

INVESTIGATIONS

- Basic observations:
  - blood pressure;
  - oxygen saturation;
  - pulse rate;
  - respiratory rate;
  - temperature.
- Blood sugar level.

DIFFERENTIAL DIAGNOSIS

- Acute head injury.
- Hypoglycaemia.
- Mixed substance misuse.

MANAGEMENT

- ABCDE approach:
  - **A**irway;
  - **B**reathing;
  - **C**irculation;
  - **D**isability;
  - **E**xposure.
- Treat any abnormalities appropriately (e.g. if hypotensive give fluids).
- Supportive management approach.

COMPLICATIONS

- Trauma or other bodily injuries.
- Haematemesis, inhalation of vomitus.
- Delirium.
- Perceptual distortions.
- Coma.

Mental health disorders

- Convulsions.
- Cardiac dysrhythmias.

PROGNOSIS

- This is a transient condition that is dose related, therefore a full recovery is expected as the substance is metabolized and excreted from the body.

5.3 HARMFUL USE

DEFINITION

- Substance misuse that has caused actual physical or mental harm to the patient.

> ## MICRO-facts
>
> **Harmful drinking**
> A pattern of drinking associated with alcohol-related harm:
>
> men > 50 units weekly;
> women > 35 units weekly.

EPIDEMIOLOGY

- 0.5–1% of people drink harmfully in the UK.

RISK FACTORS

- As for acute intoxication (see the section Acute intoxication of alcohol and other substances above).

CLINICAL FEATURES

- Physical harm:
    - liver disease/failure:
        - alcoholic liver disease,
        - hepatitis, if intravenous drug user (IVDU),
        - HIV, if IVDU;
    - local infections (IVDU), e.g. abscesses.
- Mental harm:
    - depressive disorder;
    - anxiety;
    - dementia.

INVESTIGATIONS

- Drug screen and blood alcohol level.
- Liver function tests (LFTs): raised gamma-glutamyltransferase (GGT) indicates recent alcohol intake.
- Glucose.
- Full blood count (FBC).
- Urea and electrolytes (U&E).
- B_{12} and folate.

DIFFERENTIAL DIAGNOSIS

- Substance dependence syndrome.
- Other specific drug- or alcohol-related disorders.

MANAGEMENT

- The appropriate management for the physical or mental problem.
- Address and manage the substance misuse problem appropriately.

PROGNOSIS

- The prognosis of the physical or mental problem will be problem specific.

5.4 DEPENDENCE SYNDROME

DEFINITION

- Physiological, behavioural and cognitive phenomena where the use of a substance is of greater importance than other valued behaviours.

EPIDEMIOLOGY

- In the UK 6% of men and 2% of women are alcohol dependent.

RISK FACTORS

- As for acute intoxication (see the section Acute intoxication of alcohol and other substances above).

CLINICAL FEATURES

- For diagnosis to be made at least three of the following must have been present at the same time over the past 12 months:
    - a strong desire or compulsion to take the substance;
    - problems in controlling substance taking in terms of its onset, termination or levels of use;
    - withdrawal state when the substance is removed or reduced;

Mental health disorders

- evidence of tolerance – an increasing amount of the substance must be taken to achieve the desired effect;
- neglect of other interests because of the time spent taking the substance, obtaining it or recovering from its effects;
- persisting with the substance use despite evidence of its harm.

INVESTIGATIONS

- As for those in harmful use (see the section Harmful use above).

MANAGEMENT OF ALCOHOL DEPENDENCE

- Detoxification:
  - controlled withdrawal;
  - reducing regime of a benzodiazepine;
  - encourage fluids (non-alcoholic);
  - prescribe vitamins (thiamine) as deficiencies are common;
  - can be done in the community or as an inpatient.

MICRO-facts

Detoxification

A reducing regime of chlordiazepoxide 20 mg four times a day (starting dose) to finish at a dose of 10 mg on day 5 of the detoxification is commonly used for moderate dependence.

- Maintaining abstinence:
  - abstinence – aim for abstinence rather than controlled drinking;
  - monitoring – regular LFTs and breath alcohol measurements;
  - group support – community meetings (e.g. Alcoholics Anonymous).
- Pharmacological therapy:
  - disulfiram (Antabuse) – blocks alcohol dehydrogenase so leads to an unpleasant reaction (such as flushing, tachycardia and hypotension) on drinking;
  - acamprosate [gamma-aminobutyric acid (GABA) agonist and glutamate antagonist] – reduces cravings for alcohol.
- Psychological therapy:
  - cognitive behavioural therapy;
  - motivational interviewing;
  - Alcoholics Anonymous (12-step approach);
  - social skills training.

MICRO-print

Motivational interviewing – pros and cons of drinking. Based on the model of change there are six stages:

- Pre-contemplation – not acknowledging dependence.
- Contemplation – acknowledging dependence.
- Decision.
- Action.
- Maintenance.
- Relapse.

MICRO-reference

Prochaska JO, DiClemente CC, Norcross JC. In search of how people change. Applications to addictive behaviors. *Am Psychol* 1992; **47:**1102–14.

MANAGEMENT OF OPIOID DEPENDENCE

- Detoxification:
  - inpatient detoxification is more effective than outpatient detoxification;
  - reducing regime of a substitute drug, e.g. methadone;
  - post-detoxification abstinence programmes (e.g. supportive housing).
- Maintaining abstinence:
  - aim to reduce injecting but also available are:
    - needle exchange programmes,
    - free needles and syringes;
  - stabilize drug use and lifestyle:
    - oral methadone programmes stabilize drug use and reduce the need for intravenous (IV) injections,
    - buprenorphine – can be used as an alternative to methadone;

MICRO-facts

Methadone:

- Half-life 24–36 hours.
- Starting dose is 10–30 mg per day.
- Increased by 5–10 mg per week to reach the therapeutic dose.
- Common side-effects include:
  - nausea and vomiting;
  - constipation.

Mental health disorders

- reduce criminal behaviour by reducing the use of expensive drugs;
- reduce the death rate.

COMPLICATIONS

- Can be mental or physical.
- Depends on the substance being misused.
- Alcohol related:
  - liver damage (e.g. cirrhosis and failure);
  - cardiovascular problems;
  - gastrointestinal problems;
  - Wernicke's encephalopathy;
  - Korsakoff's syndrome;
  - depression and anxiety problems;
  - suicide.
- Opioid related:
  - local damage to veins (e.g. abscesses);
  - infective endocarditis;
  - HIV;
  - hepatitis C and/or B;
  - death from overdose (respiratory failure).

PROGNOSIS

- Alcohol dependence:
  - about 50% of patients are drinking again within 6 months;
  - 30% have life-long complications;
  - 40% will die prematurely (15% suicide).
- Opioid dependence:
  - after opioid detoxification 40% will be using again at 6 months and the majority will be using again at 12 months;
  - 2–3% die annually;
  - 25% are abstinent at 5 years;
  - 40% are abstinent at 10 years.

5.5 ACUTE WITHDRAWAL STATE

See Chapter 15 Psychiatric emergencies, Acute alcohol withdrawal state with delirium.

5.6 PSYCHOTIC DISORDER ASSOCIATED WITH SUBSTANCE MISUSE

DEFINITION

- Psychotic symptoms that occur during, or immediately after substance misuse.

CLINICAL FEATURES

- Hallucinations:
  - normally auditory but may be in any sensory modality.
- Delusions:
  - paranoid or persecutory.
- Psychomotor disturbance:
  - excitement;
  - stupor.
- Abnormal affect:
  - ecstasy;
  - intense fear.
- Clouding of consciousness:
  - not severe confusion.

INVESTIGATIONS

- As for harmful use (see the section Harmful use above).

DIFFERENTIAL DIAGNOSIS

- Another mental disorder being aggravated by the substance misuse (e.g. schizophrenia).
- Paranoid or schizoid personality disorders.

MANAGEMENT

- The same as for other psychotic episodes (see Chapter 6 Schizophrenia and delusional disorders, Schizophrenia).
- Must also address and manage the cause of the psychosis.

PROGNOSIS

- It typically resolves at least partially within 1 month and fully resolves within 6 months.

5.7 WERNICKE'S ENCEPHALOPATHY AND KORSAKOFF'S SYNDROME

DEFINITION

- Memory and other cognitive impairments caused by substance misuse, most commonly alcohol.

RISK FACTORS

- The main risk factor is prolonged substance misuse (usually alcohol) which is left untreated.

PATHOPHYSIOLOGY

- Caused by damage of the mammillary bodies, hippocampus or thalamus.
- The damage is secondary to thiamine deficiency.

CLINICAL FEATURES

- Wernicke's encephalopathy:
  - memory loss;
  - ataxia;
  - ophthalmoplegia;
  - if the thiamine deficiency is not corrected, the condition may evolve into Korsakoff's syndrome.
- Korsakoff's syndrome:
  - confabulation, i.e. inaccurate recall of events with lack of insight of inaccuracy;
  - severe episodic memory problems;
  - anterograde amnesia;
  - lack of insight;
  - new learning is impaired.
- Diagnostic criteria:
  - memory impairment:
    - disturbances in recent memory,
    - disturbances in time sense (e.g. chronological sequences);
  - history or objective evidence of the chronic use of alcohol or drugs;
  - no defect in immediate recall and consciousness;
  - generalized cognitive impairment.

INVESTIGATIONS

- Thorough evaluation of cognition, e.g. mini-mental state examination (MMSE).
- LFTs.
- Thyroid function tests (TFTs).
- Syphilis serology
- Thiamine levels.
- Glucose.
- Neuroimaging to exclude other causes of dementia.

DIFFERENTIAL DIAGNOSIS

- Organic amnesic syndrome (non-alcoholic).
- Dementia.
- Delirium.
- Depression.

MANAGEMENT

- Urgent IV thiamine is required (e.g. Pabrinex).

COMPLICATIONS

- Structural complications:
  - enlarged lateral ventricles;
  - loss of cortical and subcortical grey matter;
  - thinning of the corpus callosum.
- Functional complications:
  - cognitive impairment.

MICRO-print

Korsakoff's syndrome can affect the individual's ability to self-care. Long-term rehabilitation and support may be needed.

PROGNOSIS OF KORSAKOFF'S SYNDROME

- 50% will not recover.
- 25% will partially recover.
- 25% will fully recover.

5.8 RESIDUAL AND LATE-ONSET PSYCHOTIC DISORDER

DEFINITION

- Where effects on behaviour, personality, cognition or affect are prolonged past the period where a direct psychoactive substance effect might be expected.

CLINICAL FEATURES

- Onset should be directly related to the use of alcohol or psychoactive substance.

DIFFERENTIAL DIAGNOSIS

- Pre-existing mental disorder.
- Acute and transient psychotic disorders.
- Organic injury.
- Mild or moderate mental retardation.

Mental health disorders

5.9 OTHER COMMONLY ABUSED SUBSTANCES

CANNABIS (STREET NAMES: GRASS, POT)

- Effects:
  - euphoria and disinhibition;
  - anxiety or agitation;
  - suspiciousness or paranoid ideation;
  - slowing in time;
  - impaired judgement, attention or reaction time;
  - auditory, visual or tactile illusions;
  - hallucinations with preserved orientation;
  - depersonalization or derealization;
  - interface with personal functioning.
- Signs:
  - increased appetite;
  - dry mouth;
  - conjunctival injection (reddening of eyes);
  - tachycardia.
- Complications:
  - chronic amotivational syndrome;
  - impaired concentration;
  - paranoia;
  - anxiety.

METHYLENEDIOXYMETHAMPHETAMINE (MDMA; STREET NAME: ECSTASY)

- Effects:
  - tachycardia;
  - dry mouth;
  - jaw clenching;
  - muscle aches;
  - increased alertness;
  - lasts 4–6 hours.
- Complications:
  - hyperthermia syndrome (nausea, sweating and palpitation);
  - convulsion;
  - sudden death.

COCAINE (STREET NAME: COKE)

- Effects:
  - stimulant;
  - increased alertness;

- confidence;
- short duration;
- involuntary motor activity;
- stereotyped behaviour;
- paranoia.
- Complications:
  - withdrawal (e.g. fatigue, depression);
  - cardiac arrhythmias;
  - palpitations and chest pain;
  - convulsions;
  - overdose.

CRACK COCAINE (STREET NAMES: ROCK, STONE)

- Effects:
  - stimulant;
  - euphoria;
  - lasts about 10 minutes.
- Complications:
  - highly addictive;
  - cardiac problems;
  - afterwards – paranoia, psychosis and confusion.

LYSERGIC ACID DIETHYLAMIDE (LSD; STREET NAMES: TRIPS, ACID)

- Effects:
  - hallucinogenic;
  - stimulation of one sense stimulates sensation in the other sense (e.g. intense experience of 'hearing' the colour);
  - effects vary depending on the users mood;
  - lasts 8–12 hours.
- Complications:
  - bad 'trip' – anxiety, paranoia, feeling out of control;
  - accidents;
  - flashbacks.

MAGIC MUSHROOMS

- Effects:
  - similar to LSD;
  - relaxation;
  - lasts about 4 hours.
- Complications:
  - abdominal pain;
  - sickness and diarrhoea.

Mental health disorders

SOLVENT (E.G. GLUE)

- Effects:
  - apathy and lethargy;
  - argumentativeness;
  - abusiveness or aggression;
  - lability of mood;
  - impaired attention and memory;
  - impaired judgement;
  - psychomotor retardation;
  - interference with personal functioning.
- Signs:
  - unsteady gait;
  - difficulty in standing;
  - slurred speech;
  - decreased conscious level;
  - nystagmus;
  - muscle weakness;
  - blurred vision or diplopia.
- Complications:
  - change in personality;
  - cognitive impairment;
  - nasal septum perforation.

MICRO-print
Legal highs
There is a new and growing trend for people to achieve euphoric states through the use of a variety of substances which are currently not banned under UK law as being illicit drugs. These compounds are sold in 'head shops' and widely over the Internet. Under current medicines legislation, these compounds would be illegal to advertise or sell for human consumption and they are therefore marketed as 'plant food', 'cleaning products', etc. Examples include 'Bubble' (amphetamine-like properties) and methoxetamine (also called MXE, MKET or Roflcoptr).

---

6 Schizophrenia and delusional disorders

6.1 SCHIZOPHRENIA

> **MICRO-case**
>
> Mr X is a 35-year-old unemployed man admitted to the psychiatric ward under Section 2 of the Mental Health Act. He has a 6-month history of increasingly isolating himself. His friends have noticed that whenever they see him he is 'not quite right' and he constantly appears to be talking to himself. Before admission he vandalized his flat, which he shares with his girlfriend and was both verbally and physically aggressive towards her. On assessment by the house officer he states that he has been hearing 'nasty voices' which have been telling him to do things, e.g. that he should 'smash up his flat' and to hurt himself and others. He admits to having tried to kill himself, 'using his thoughts'; however, when this didn't work he became very angry. Mr X says that he is concerned that recently he had not felt as if his thoughts were private and that if he was walking around on the streets, then anyone within 10 m of him could hear what he was thinking. This has led to him barricading himself in his flat where he has remained for the past fortnight. He denies any drug or alcohol use or any medical problems.
>
> **Learning points**
>
> - Psychotic symptoms can cause marked changes in perception.
> - Psychosis can have a significant impact on both the patient and the people in the patient's life.

EPIDEMIOLOGY

- 1-year incidence rate: 15–50 per 100 000.
- Point prevalence: 1%.
- Lifetime risk: 1%.
- Age of onset: between 15 years and 45 years.
- Male to female ratio: 1:1.
- Women tend to have a later age of onset.
- Symptoms in men tend to be more severe.

> ## MICRO-facts
>
> ### Social drift
> Having a diagnosis of schizophrenia makes it more likely that you, and therefore your children, will 'drift' down the social classes as a result of impaired social functioning and inability to cope – the so-called **social drift.** This makes it difficult to decide if low social class is caused by schizophrenia or is an effect of the course and nature of the illness.

- Epidemiological risk factors:
  - being unmarried;
  - being an immigrant (e.g. Afro-Caribbean immigrants);
  - living in an urban area;
  - lower social class.

AETIOLOGY

> ## MICRO-facts
>
> There has been much research into the development of schizophrenia which has implicated genes, biochemical abnormalities and environmental triggers as possible aetiological factors. The fact that the concordance rate for **monozygotic twins** is not 100% (in fact it is only about 45%) and that some individuals develop the disorder without anyone in the family suffering from it, suggests a highly complex **multifactorial** pathogenesis that is not entirely understood.

- Genetic factors:
  - family studies:
    - ~10% chance of developing schizophrenia if a first-degree relative has it,
    - ~50% chance of developing schizophrenia if both parents have it,
    - the more family members affected, the greater the chance an individual has of developing the illness.

> ### MICRO-print
> There is a proposed link between development of schizophrenia and babies born to older fathers. It has been suggested that an increased likelihood of gene mutation can account for this.

- twin studies:
  - ~10% chance in dizygotic twins,
  - ~45% chance in monozygotic twins;
- adoption studies:
  - ~10% chance of developing schizophrenia if a biological parent has it;
- cannabis use may increase the risk of schizophrenia in people who are homozygous for Val/Val alleles in COMT genotypes.

MICRO-print

There has been some evidence to suggest the genes *DTNBP1* (dystrobrevin binding protein 1) on chromosome 6p22.3, *NRG1* (neuregulin 1) on chromosome 8p21–22 and chromosome 22q11 (velo-cardio-facial syndrome), among others, have a part to play in the aetiology of schizophrenia.

Data from Norton N, Williams HJ, Owen MJ. An update on the genetics of schizophrenia. *Current Opinion in Psychiatry* 2006; **19**: 158–64.

- Prenatal and perinatal factors:
  - increased risk of schizophrenia in adults who were born during winter and early spring (increased risk of maternal influenza infection);
  - increased risk of schizophrenia in adults born to mothers who had measles or rubella during pregnancy;
  - increased risk of early-onset schizophrenia in males who were small for gestational age, those whose mothers had antenatal bleeds and in those born to multiparous women.
- Neurodevelopmental theory:
  - genetic, prenatal and perinatal risk factors cause a disturbance in which the normal pattern of programmed cell death is compromised, leading to a defect in the normal orderly migration of neurons toward the cortical plate; this has serious consequences for the establishment of a normal pattern of cortical connections;
  - constellation of early signs in childhood include abnormal eye (saccadic) tracking movements, neuropsychological deficits, soft neurological signs [e.g. clumsiness, incoordination or non-specific electroencephalogram (EEG) changes] and abnormal behaviours;
  - classical schizophrenia symptoms do not appear because the brain is not fully developed;
  - classical schizophrenia symptoms emerge in young adulthood as a result of accumulated intracerebral pathology and spatial disarray of neurons in a mature human brain.

Mental health disorders

- Home environment:
  - stressful life events within the month preceding onset can trigger the first schizophrenic episode in predisposed individuals;
  - high levels of expressed emotion (i.e. high levels of anger, blame, intolerance and intrusion into person's life) within the home can cause relapse in a patient with schizophrenia;
  - increased risk of schizophrenia in children where there are a large number of siblings (increased risk of infection in early infancy).
- Neuroanatomical abnormalities:
  - findings on structural neuroimaging:
    - lateral and third ventricular enlargement,
    - atrophy of prefrontal cortex and temporal lobe,
    - smaller thalamus,
    - enlarged caudate nucleus,
    - reduction in overall brain volume.
- Neurotransmitter abnormalities:
  - dopamine hypothesis: this states that schizophrenia is the result of dopaminergic hyperactivity in the mesolimbic–mesocortical pathway;
  - evidence in support of the dopamine hypothesis:
    - antipsychotics are dopamine D_2 receptor antagonists and cause a reduction in the positive symptoms of schizophrenia,
    - drugs that increase cerebral dopamine levels (e.g. amphetamines) can cause psychosis;
  - serotonin: excess serotonin has been linked to schizophrenia;
  - evidence in support of serotonin's involvement in schizophrenia:
    - the antipsychotic risperidone is a potent 5-hydroxytryptamine receptor ($5HT_2$) antagonist,
    - clozapine is very effective in treatment resistant schizophrenia and has an affinity for $5HT_2$ and $5HT_3$ receptors while binding only weakly to D_2 receptors,
    - drugs that increase cerebral serotonin levels such as LSD (lysergic acid diethylamide) can induce psychotic symptoms.

CLINICAL FEATURES

In the ICD-10, five main subtypes of schizophrenia can be distinguished based on their characteristics and course (see Fig. 6.1 for symptoms).

> **MICRO-reference**
> http://apps.who.int/classifications/icd10/browse/2010/en

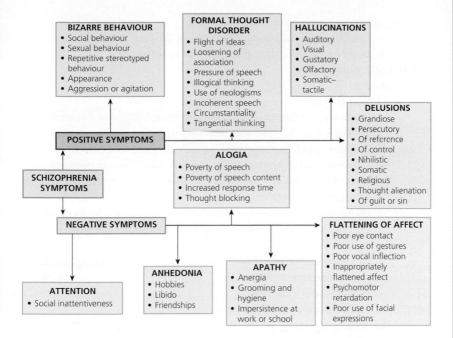

Fig. 6.1 Symptoms of schizophrenia.

- Paranoid schizophrenia:
  - most common type;
  - clinical features:
    - paranoid delusions (delusions of persecution/reference/control),
    - auditory hallucinations (second- or third-person),
    - perceptual disturbance,
    - hallucinations of smell, taste, sexual or other bodily sensations;
  - course and prognosis:
    - later onset of illness,
    - better prognosis than other types.
- Hebephrenic schizophrenia:
  - clinical features:
    - disorganized thinking and incoherent speech,
    - shallow, often inappropriate mood,
    - prominent changes of volition and affect (incongruent or flat),
    - irresponsible and unpredictable behaviour,
    - delusions and hallucinations are fleeting and fragmentary,
    - mannerisms are common;

- course and prognosis:
  - usually occurs in young adults under 25 years,
  - poorer prognosis than paranoid schizophrenia.
- Catatonic schizophrenia:
  - rare;
  - clinical features:
    - psychomotor disturbance prominent – can alternate between extremes (e.g. hyperkinesis and stupor),
    - catatonic rigidity,
    - catatonic posturing (maintains inappropriate/bizarre postures),
    - catatonic negativism (motiveless resistance to instructions or attempts to be moved),
    - catatonic waxy flexibility (flexibilitas cerea: patient's limbs retain the position into which they were placed by another person),
    - catatonic excitement (purposeless motor activity),
    - catatonic stupor (decreased reactivity to environment, spontaneous movement and activity),
    - echopraxia or echolalia,
    - mannerisms, stereotypies and tics.
- Residual schizophrenia:
  - 1-year history of negative symptoms following an episode of one of the above types of schizophrenia;
  - clinical features:
    - blunting of affect,
    - psychomotor slowing,
    - passivity,
    - poverty of speech,
    - poor eye contact,
    - poor facial movement,
    - underactivity,
    - poor self-care,
    - poor voice modulation,
    - poor posture.
- Simple schizophrenia:
  - uncommon;
  - insidious but progressive development of odd conduct and decline in performance;
  - negative symptoms of residual schizophrenia without a preceding typical schizophrenic episode;
  - clinical features:
    - as residual schizophrenia (above),
    - inability to meet demands of society.

MICRO-facts

Use the following mnemonic to remember the subtypes:

People (paranoid)
Hear (hebephrenic)
Running (residual)
Commentaries (catatonic)
in **S**chizophrenia (simple)

MICRO-print

DSM-IV-TR criteria for schizophrenia differ from the ICD-10 in the following ways:

- Hebephrenic and simple schizophrenia are not present in the DSM-IV-TR.
- Social and occupation disturbance must last for at least 6 months with at least 1 month of schizophrenic symptoms.
- Schizophreniform disorder (disturbance between 1 and 6 months) and brief psychotic disorder (less than 1 month) are found in the DSM-IV-TR but not in the ICD-10.

MICRO-reference

American Psychiatric Association. *Diagnostic and statistical manual of mental disorders*, 4th edn (text revision). Washington, DC: American Psychiatric Association, 2000.

- Schneider's first-rank symptoms:
  - one or more of these symptoms makes the diagnosis of schizophrenia more likely:
    - delusional perception – of a normal stimulus (e.g. person hears the phone ring and immediately knows that the Prime Minister's life is in danger),
    - thought alienation (i.e. thought insertion/withdrawal/broadcast),
    - passivity phenomena (i.e. made actions/feelings/thoughts),
    - auditory hallucinations (second- or third-person: thought echo, running commentary, voices discussing patient).
- Other important symptoms from the ICD-10:
  - negative symptoms;
  - circumstantiality;
  - tangentiality;
  - loosening of association (derailment/neologisms/word salad);

- flight of ideas (clang/pun associations);
- thought blocking;
- perseveration;
- echolalia;
- irrelevant ideas.

SCREENING QUESTIONS

- Hallucinations:
    - Do you ever hear strange noises that others can't hear? (**auditory** hallucinations);
    - Do you ever hear voices that no one else can hear? (**auditory** hallucinations);
    - Do you ever hear your own thoughts echoed after you think them? (**thought echo**);
    - Do the voices you hear talk to you or tell you to do anything? (**second-person auditory** hallucinations/command);
    - How many voices do you hear? (**third-person auditory** hallucinations);
    - Do the voices you hear talk to each other or give a running commentary of your actions? (**third-person auditory** hallucinations);
    - What sort of things do the voices say? (determining congruency of **auditory** hallucinations);
    - Do you ever see things that others don't see? (**visual** hallucinations);
    - Do you smell or taste things that cannot be readily explained? (**olfactory/gustatory** hallucinations).
- Delusions:
    - Do you feel that there are people trying to harm or kill you? (delusions of **persecution**);
    - Do you ever think that the TV or radio send special messages directed specifically at you? (delusions of **reference**);
    - Do you have any special powers or abilities that others don't have? (delusions of **grandeur**);
    - Do you feel like you deserve punishment for mistakes you made in the past? Can you tell me the nature of the mistakes and punishment you deserve? (delusions of **guilt**);
    - Do you feel like you no longer exist/the world no longer exists/the world is about to cease to exist? (**nihilistic** delusion).
- Thought alienation:
    - Do you feel as if something or someone is putting thoughts into your head? (thought **insertion**);
    - Do you feel as if there are people accessing and removing your thoughts? (thought **withdrawal**);
    - Do you feel as if someone or something is causing your thoughts to be heard out loud by others? (thought **broadcast**).

- Passivity phenomena:
  - Do you feel as if you are being made to do things out of your control by an external force? (made **actions**);
  - Do you feel as if your emotions are being controlled? (made **emotions**);
  - Do you feel as if your thoughts are being controlled? (made **thoughts**).
- Assess negative symptoms:
  - Do you encounter any difficulty in looking after yourself? (**apathy**);
  - How often do you tend to take a shower or a bath? (**apathy**);
  - Is it difficult to stay tidy or to keep your house clean? (**apathy**);
  - Have you spent any time with friends or family members lately? (**anhedonia**);
  - Do you find it difficult to feel close emotionally to other people? (**anhedonia**);
  - Do you have any activity you enjoy nowadays? (**anhedonia**).
- Assess insight:
  - What do you think is the cause for these experiences?
  - Could you be suffering from a mental illness?
  - Would you be willing to accept treatment to reduce these experiences?

INVESTIGATIONS

- Schizophrenia is a clinical diagnosis; therefore, investigations are aimed at excluding medical conditions or substance abuse as a cause of the psychosis (Table 6.1).
- It is important to get a collateral history from a family member or the patient's general practitioner (GP) to ensure that you have complete and accurate information about the patient's usual behaviours and premorbid personality.
- Bloods:
  - full blood count (FBC):
    - to exclude delirium as a cause of psychosis (e.g. raised white cell count),
    - for baseline check,
    - essential if starting clozapine (risk of agranulocytosis);
  - urea and electrolytes (U&E): for baseline check as most antipsychotics are excreted renally;
  - liver function tests (LFTs): for baseline check as some antipsychotics are excreted by the liver (e.g. clozapine);
  - thyroid function tests (TFTs): to exclude thyroid disorders as a cause of psychosis;
  - serum calcium and parathyroid hormone (PTH): to exclude parathyroid dysfunction as a cause of psychosis;
  - syphilis screen: to exclude neurosyphilis as a cause of psychosis (if suspected);

Mental health disorders

Table 6.1 Differential diagnoses for schizophrenia.

MEDICAL CONDITIONS	SUBSTANCE ABUSE
Neurological disease: Huntington's disease, temporal lobe epilepsy, brain tumours, HIV, CJD, neurosyphilis, head trauma, stroke, dementia	Stimulants: amphetamine, cocaine, ecstasy, caffeine
Endocrine disease: hyper/ hypothyroidism, hyperparathyroidism, Cushing's disease	Hallucinogens: LSD, magic mushrooms (psilocybin)
Vitamin deficiencies: vitamin B_{12}, thiamine (Wernicke's encephalopathy), niacin	Inhalants: glue, aerosols, paint, petrol
Others: SLE, acute intermittent porphyria, delirium	Medications: corticosteroids, anticholinergics, antiparkinsonian drugs
	Others: alcohol withdrawal, cannabis

CJD, Creutzfeldt–Jakob disease; HIV, human immunodeficiency virus; LSD, lysergic acid diethylamide; SLE, systemic lupus erythematosus.

- vitamin B_{12}: to exclude vitamin B_{12} deficiency as a cause of psychosis;
- human immunodeficiency virus (HIV) screen: to exclude HIV as a cause of psychosis (if suspected).
- Urine toxicology screen: to exclude substance abuse as a cause of psychosis.
- Electrocardiogram (ECG): for baseline check (many antipsychotics cause QT prolongation).
- EEG: to exclude temporal lobe epilepsy as cause of psychosis (if suspected).
- Computed tomography (CT)/magnetic resonance imaging (MRI): to exclude space occupying lesion (cerebral abscess, subdural haematoma, brain tumour) or vasculitis as cause of psychosis (if suspected).

MANAGEMENT

- No known cure.
- Treatment is aimed at reducing symptoms, preventing relapse and preventing chronic disability.
- First episode:
  - early referral to psychiatric services in secondary care is essential;
  - may need hospitalization for assessment and instigation of treatment;

- first-line treatment:
  - atypical antipsychotic such as olanzapine to reduce likelihood of extrapyramidal side-effects associated with older (typical) antipsychotics,
  - start at low dose and titrate upwards,
  - choice of drug should be patient-centred and based on discussion around side-effects and monitoring, etc.,
  - trial for at least 2 weeks, ideally 6–8 weeks to assess effectiveness;
- give antipsychotics for 2 years with regular reviews; up to 80% relapse if antipsychotics are stopped early (<1 year).
- Acute episode:
  - may need hospitalization if psychosis is likely to lead to harm of patient or others;
  - consider rapid tranquilization if the patient is aggressive or posing a threat to themselves or others:
    - accepting oral medication:
      - lorazepam 1–2 mg if patient is already on an oral antipsychotic,
      - an oral atypical antipsychotic (e.g. olanzapine 10 mg) or a typical drug (e.g. haloperidol 5 mg) if the patient is not already on an antipsychotic;
    - refusing oral medication:
      - intramuscular (IM) lorazepam 1–2 mg,
      - ± IM haloperidol 5–10 mg,
      - IM olanzapine 10 mg can be given instead of haloperidol but **never** at the same time as IM benzodiazepines (risk of severe hypotension and sedation).

MICRO-facts

The majority of antipsychotics are ineffective against negative symptoms; however, low-dose amisulpride has been shown to be effective in these patients.

- Relapse/multiple episodes:
  - give antipsychotics long term with regular reviews;
  - if compliance is likely to be an issue, then depot injection of several typical antipsychotics are available which only need to be given once every few weeks e.g. zuclopenthixol decanoate. Atypical drugs are not commonly available in depot form, except risperidone and more recently olanzapine and paliperidone.
- Psychological therapy:
  - cognitive behavioural therapy (CBT) should be offered to all patients;

- family intervention:
  - to reduce expressed emotion and negative home atmosphere (associated with increased relapse rates);
- social skills training;
- occupational therapy to help patients with skills such as cooking.
- Follow-up:
  - patients should be followed up in the community by the community psychiatric team;
  - after discharge from any hospitalization patients should be seen by a psychiatrist in the community as often as clinically indicated.

PROGNOSIS

- ~25% of patients have one single episode and go on to have a good long-term outcome.
- ~50% have significant morbidity with multiple relapses and recurrent hospitalizations (see Table 6.2).

Table 6.2 Prognostic indicators in schizophrenia.

	GOOD PROGNOSTIC FACTORS	POOR PROGNOSTIC FACTORS
Patient demographics	Female Married	Male Unmarried
Aetiology	Precipitated by stressful life events No past psychiatric history Family history of affective illness	Past psychiatric history Family history of schizophrenia
Nature of illness	Late onset of symptoms Paranoid type Positive symptoms	Early onset of symptoms Negative symptoms
Treatment	Good response Short duration of untreated psychosis	Poor response Long duration of untreated psychosis

6.2 DELUSIONAL DISORDERS

MICRO-case

Mr Z is a 45-year-old married man with no past psychiatric history. He has been married for 20 years and has always been 'the jealous type'; however, he has recently become convinced that his wife is having an affair after she started attending evening art classes. At first this was just a niggling thought, but it has since turned into an obsession that he says has been keeping him awake at night. He admits to rooting through the laundry basket on nights that she has been out to try and find any evidence of her infidelity. Last week he confronted Mrs Z about his suspicions. She became very upset about his accusations and they had a blistering row ending in him hitting her.

Learning points

- Delusions of jealousy can interfere with normal home life and become very distressing for all persons involved.

EPIDEMIOLOGY

- Incidence rate: 1–3 per 100 000.
- Point prevalence: 0.03%.
- Lifetime risk: 0.05–0.1%.
- Mean age of onset: 35 years for men, 45 years for women.
- Male to female ratio: male < female (slight).
- Men are more likely to develop paranoid delusions.
- Women are more likely to develop delusions of erotomania.

AETIOLOGY

- Genetic factors:
  - increased incidence of delusional disorder in patients who have a first-degree relative with schizophrenia;
  - increased incidence of paranoid personality disorder in patients who have a first-degree relative with delusional disorder (not applicable to any of the other personality disorders).
- Neuroanatomical abnormalities:
  - in the basal ganglia (excess dopamine);
  - in the limbic system.
- Psychological factors:
  - neuropsychological models:

Mental health disorders

- – cognitive bias model (CBM) – paranoid delusions are a defence mechanism to protect self from thoughts that threaten a person's self-image,
  - – cognitive deficit model (CDM) – delusions are caused by cognitive impairments and a misinterpretation of external reality.
- Organic conditions that can cause psychosis:
  - neurological disease (multiple sclerosis, Alzheimer's disease, Parkinson's disease, Huntington's disease, brain tumours, epilepsy, Pick's disease, fat embolism);
  - vascular disease (subarachnoid haemorrhage, atherosclerosis, hypertensive encephalopathy, temporal arteritis);
  - infectious disease [HIV, acquired immune deficiency syndrome (AIDS), Creutzfeldt–Jakob disease (CJD), syphilis, malaria, acute viral encephalitis];
  - metabolic disorder (hypercalcaemia, hyponatraemia, hypoglycaemia, uraemia, hepatic encephalopathy, acute intermittent porphyria);
  - endocrinopathies (Addison's disease, Cushing's syndrome, hypothyroidism, hyperthyroidism, panhypopituitarism);
  - vitamin deficiencies (vitamin B_{12}, folate, thiamine, niacin).

CLINICAL FEATURES

- ICD-10 criteria for diagnosing delusional disorders:
  - delusion/set of delusions other than those listed as typically schizophrenic (i.e. not delusions of control, delusions of passivity, delusional perceptions);
  - delusions lasting ≥ 3 months;
  - other criteria of schizophrenia are not filled (remember the first-rank symptoms);
  - no persistent hallucinations, although transitory hallucinations may be a feature (especially in elderly patients);
  - no mood disturbances occurring simultaneously to delusions (depressive symptoms may occur intermittently);
  - no evidence of organic or psychotic disorder, or psychoactive substance abuse disorder.
- The delusion is persistent and can sometimes be lifelong.
- The DSM-IV-TR states that the delusions are non-bizarre delusions and involve situations that occur in real life (e.g. being followed, deceived by a spouse, having a disease, being infected or poisoned).
- You can classify delusional disorders into subtypes depending on their features (Fig. 6.2).

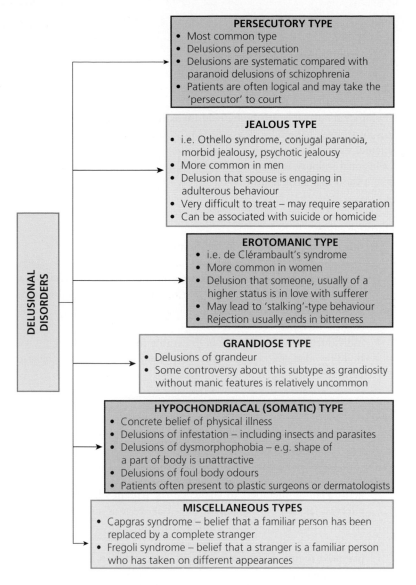

PERSECUTORY TYPE
- Most common type
- Delusions of persecution
- Delusions are systematic compared with paranoid delusions of schizophrenia
- Patients are often logical and may take the 'persecutor' to court

JEALOUS TYPE
- i.e. Othello syndrome, conjugal paranoia, morbid jealousy, psychotic jealousy
- More common in men
- Delusion that spouse is engaging in adulterous behaviour
- Very difficult to treat – may require separation
- Can be associated with suicide or homicide

EROTOMANIC TYPE
- i.e. de Clérambault's syndrome
- More common in women
- Delusion that someone, usually of a higher status is in love with sufferer
- May lead to 'stalking'-type behaviour
- Rejection usually ends in bitterness

GRANDIOSE TYPE
- Delusions of grandeur
- Some controversy about this subtype as grandiosity without manic features is relatively uncommon

HYPOCHONDRIACAL (SOMATIC) TYPE
- Concrete belief of physical illness
- Delusions of infestation – including insects and parasites
- Delusions of dysmorphophobia – e.g. shape of a part of body is unattractive
- Delusions of foul body odours
- Patients often present to plastic surgeons or dermatologists

MISCELLANEOUS TYPES
- Capgras syndrome – belief that a familiar person has been replaced by a complete stranger
- Fregoli syndrome – belief that a stranger is a familiar person who has taken on different appearances

DELUSIONAL DISORDERS

Fig. 6.2 Features and classification of delusional disorders.

INVESTIGATIONS

- It is important to initially **confirm** the diagnosis of delusional disorder.
- Bloods to exclude medical causes (see the section on Schizophrenia above):
  - LFTs;
  - U&E;

- vitamin B_{12} and folate;
- TFTs;
- serum calcium and PTH levels;
- syphilis screen;
- HIV test;
- malaria blood film.
- Owing to abnormal beliefs being held incredibly strongly (hence delusional), it is imperative that a full risk assessment is done, including risk of self-harm, suicide, violence, aggression and homicide.
- Delusional jealousy is common in alcoholics; therefore, it is important to take a thorough alcohol history.

MANAGEMENT

- Hospitalization:
  - this may be appropriate in the following circumstances:
    - ideas of suicide or self-harm,
    - ideas of violence or aggression or hurting others,
    - detention under the Mental Health Act may be needed to protect the patient and/or others.
- Psychological therapy:
  - individual cognitive therapy is preferable to group therapy;
  - building adequate rapport with the patient is important to reverse delusional ideas;

> **MICRO-facts**
>
> The therapist should initially neither agree nor disagree with the patient's delusions. This helps to establish **rapport**.

  - getting family members to challenge the patient's beliefs can be very effective (as long as the patient does not see it as an attempt to side with the therapist – therefore tread carefully!).
- Pharmacological therapy:
  - paranoid symptoms are treated with antipsychotics just as in schizophrenia;
  - non-sedating and newer antipsychotics (better tolerability) are preferred.
- Co-morbid depressive symptoms are treated with antidepressants as usual if required.

6.3 ACUTE AND TRANSIENT PSYCHOTIC DISORDERS

EPIDEMIOLOGY

- Uncommon.
- Male to female ratio: male < female.
- Age of onset: 20–30 years.
- Age of onset is higher in industrialized settings.
- Associated with certain personality disorders: histrionic, paranoid, borderline, narcissistic and schizotypal.
- More commonly seen in people who have faced major disasters or cultural change and those from lower social classes.

AETIOLOGY

- Tentative link with a family history of mood disorders or schizophrenia.
- Acute psychosocial stressors such as bereavement or the psychological trauma of war can trigger onset.

CLINICAL FEATURES

- Sudden change of a person's mental state from normal to psychotic.
- It can be hard to diagnose this disorder because of features that mimic other psychoses; therefore, the ICD-10 states a diagnostic sequence depending on the importance of the criterion:
  - an acute onset (within 2 weeks) as the defining feature of the whole group;
  - the presence of typical syndromes;
  - the presence of associated stress.

> ## MICRO-facts
>
> ### ICD-10 diagnostic criteria
>
> - Psychotic mental state that does not meet the criteria for schizophrenia.
> - Does not satisfy criteria for manic or depressive episode (although emotional changes and individual affective symptoms may be prominent from time to time).
> - Absence of organic cause (e.g. concussion, delirium, dementia) or intoxication by drugs or alcohol.
>
> *continued...*

Mental health disorders

continued...

- The 2 week window of development of the disorder describes the time to when the symptoms become obvious and disruptive of at least some aspects of daily life and work.
- Psychotic state can be classified as either without associated acute stress or with associated acute stress.

- Onset is said to be abrupt if the psychotic state occurs within 48 hours.
- There are a number of typical syndromes as described by the ICD-10:
- Acute polymorphic psychotic disorder without symptoms of schizophrenia:
  - several types of hallucination or delusion;
  - hallucinations/delusions change in type and intensity from day to day or within the same day;
  - emotional state is similarly variable;
  - symptoms are not present with sufficient consistency to fulfil the criteria for either schizophrenia, manic episode or depressive episode.

MICRO-facts

The term 'polymorphic' here describes the great variability seen in these patients' emotions and psychotic symptoms.

- Acute polymorphic psychotic disorder with symptoms of schizophrenia:
  - several types of hallucination or delusion;
  - hallucinations/delusions change in type and intensity from day to day or within the same day;
  - emotional state is similarly variable;
  - symptoms fulfil the criteria for schizophrenia and have been present for the majority of time since the onset of the psychotic state;
  - if schizophrenic symptoms last >1 month the diagnosis should be changed to schizophrenia.
- Acute schizophrenia-like psychotic disorder:
  - psychotic symptoms are relatively stable;
  - symptoms fulfil the criteria for schizophrenia;
  - symptoms last <1 month;
  - may be some degree of emotional variability;
  - if schizophrenic symptoms last >1 month the diagnosis should be changed to schizophrenia.
- Other acute and predominantly delusional psychotic disorders:
  - relatively stable hallucinations or delusions;
  - delusions or hallucinations must have been present for the majority of the time since the onset of the psychotic state;

- symptoms do not fulfil the criteria for schizophrenia or acute polymorphic psychotic disorder;
- if delusions last >3 months the diagnosis should be changed to persistent delusional disorder;
- if hallucinations last >3 months the diagnosis should be changed to other non-organic psychotic disorder.
- Diagnosing the subtype in a patient with an acute psychotic state: see Fig. 6.3.

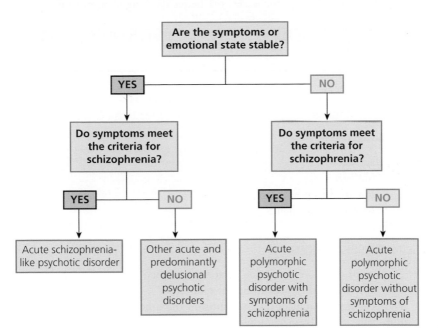

Fig. 6.3 Classification of acute and transient psychotic disorders.

MANAGEMENT

- Hospitalization (if needed for the safety of the patient or others) is usually brief.
- Psychological therapy:
    - use of psychotherapy to help the patient understand and accept the psychotic episode as well as explore possible triggers;
    - psychotherapy where the patient's family have an active involvement is associated with a better prognosis.
- Pharmacological therapy:
    - short-term use of antipsychotic (e.g. haloperidol) to control psychosis but beware of extrapyramidal side-effects;

Mental health disorders

- short-term use of benzodiazepine (e.g. lorazepam) – fewer side-effects than antipsychotics, therefore tolerated better;
- avoid long-term drug use as these are short-lived episodes.

PROGNOSIS

- Complete recovery usually occurs within 2–3 months.
- A small proportion will go on to have chronic symptoms.
- Relapse is common.
- The more acute/abrupt the onset, the better the long-term outcome.

6.4 INDUCED DELUSIONAL DISORDER (FOLIE À DEUX)

EPIDEMIOLOGY

- Very rare disorder.

AETIOLOGY

- Risk factors:
  - old age;
  - low intelligence;
  - sensory impairment;
  - alcohol abuse.

CLINICAL FEATURES

- Transfer of delusions from one person to another.
- Delusions are usually persecutory or grandiose.
- The person who induces the delusions on the other is usually the more dominant within their relationship.
- The persons involved are often isolated from others either geographically, by culture or language.

MICRO-facts

ICD-10 diagnostic criteria:

- 2 or more people share the same delusion or delusional disorder and **support** each other in this belief.
- The persons have an unusually close relationship.
- There is **temporal** or other **contextual** evidence that the delusion was induced in the passive member(s) of the pair or group by contact with the active member.

MANAGEMENT

- Separation of the persons usually reverses delusions in the passive individual.
- Hospitalization may be indicated if risk of self-harm/harm to others.
- Pharmacological therapy:
    - as for other delusional disorders, but the potential for side-effects must be carefully explored: patients with induced delusional disorders tend to be older;
    - atypical antipsychotic (e.g. aripiprazole or quetiapine) may be better tolerated.

6.5 SCHIZOAFFECTIVE DISORDERS

EPIDEMIOLOGY

- Lifetime prevalence (estimated): <1% (0.05–0.08%).
- Male to female ratio: male < female.

MICRO-facts

Older patients are more likely to suffer from **depressive type**, whereas younger patients are more likely to have **bipolar type**.

- Women tend to have a later age of onset (as for schizophrenia).

AETIOLOGY

- Unclear.
- Some evidence of a genetic basis.

MICRO-print

A gene on chromosome 1q42 close to the *DISC1* gene has been linked to schizoaffective disorder.

MICRO-reference

Hamshere ML, Bennett P, Williams N, Segurado R, Cardno A, Norton N et al. Genome-wide linkage scan in schizoaffective disorder: significant evidence for linkage at 1q42 close to DISC1, and suggestive evidence at 22q11 and 19p13. *Arch Gen Psychiatry* 2005; **62:** 1081–8.

Mental health disorders

CLINICAL FEATURES

- Schizophrenic **and** affective symptoms are prominent.
- The schizophrenic and affective symptoms should either occur simultaneously or within a few days of each other, but within the same episode.
- The ICD-10 classifies schizoaffective disorder depending on the affect of the person – the main 3 subtypes are shown in Fig. 6.4.

SCHIZOAFFECTIVE DISORDER: MANIC TYPE
- **Manic symptoms:** e.g. elation, excitement, irritability, aggression, over-activity, increased energy, flight of ideas, impaired concentration, grandiose ideas
- **Psychotic symptoms:** e.g. thought alienation, passivity phenomena, delusions of persecution or reference and third-person auditory hallucinations
- Presents as an acute florid psychosis

SCHIZOAFFECTIVE DISORDER: DEPRESSIVE TYPE
- **Depressive symptoms:** e.g. low mood, psychomotor retardation, insomnia, anergia, anhedonia, decreased appetite, weight loss, impaired concentration, guilt, feelings of hopelessness and suicidal thoughts
- **Psychotic symptoms** (see above)
- Usually lasts longer than manic type
- Less alarming presentation than manic type

SCHIZOAFFECTIVE DISORDER: MIXED TYPE
- **Psychotic symptoms** (see above)
- Symptoms of **bipolar affective disorder, current episode mixed,** e.g. low mood, anergia and loss of libido alternating rapidly with manic mood, grandiosity, agitation, overactivity and pressure of speech, or a mixture of these symptoms during the episode

Fig. 6.4 Features and classification of schizoaffective disorder.

INVESTIGATIONS

- To exclude organic causes of the symptoms (see the section on Schizophrenia above):
  - FBC;
  - U&E;

- LFTs;
- TFTs;
- serum calcium and PTH;
- syphilis screen;
- vitamin B$_{12}$;
- urine drug screen;
- HIV screen;
- ECG;
- EEG;
- CT/MRI.
- You need to exclude other psychiatric disorders:
  - bipolar affective disorder;
  - schizophrenia;
  - depression with psychotic features.

MANAGEMENT

- Hospitalization:
  - if risk of self-harm, suicide or self-neglect;
  - if risk to others.
- Psychological therapy:
  - family therapy is very important for these disorders;
  - social skills training (as for schizophrenia);
  - cognitive rehabilitation;
  - patient and family education can help hugely as this is a chronic disorder, so early recognition of signs and symptoms is useful.
- Pharmacological therapy:
  - atypical antipsychotics are usually used to treat psychotic symptoms;
  - manic subtype:
    - mood stabilizer, e.g. lithium or carbamazepine;
  - depressive subtype:
    - antidepressant, usually a selective serotonin re-uptake inhibitor (SSRI) such as fluoxetine;
  - treatment resistant:
    - electroconvulsive therapy (ECT).

PROGNOSIS

- Long-term outcome is better than schizophrenia, but worse than affective disorders.
- Manic subtype has a better prognosis than depressive subtype.
- A full recovery usually occurs within weeks in manic subtype.

Mental health disorders

Affective disorders

7.1 MANIC EPISODE

EPIDEMIOLOGY

- Prevalence (estimated): 0.4–1.6%.
- Age of onset: peaks in early adult life.
- Male to female ratio: 1:1.

AETIOLOGY

- Genetic factors:
  - twin studies:
    - ~ 65–75% concordance in monozygotic twins,
    - ~ 14% concordance in dizygotic twins.
- Neurotransmitter abnormalities:
  - monoamine theory: increased levels of noradrenaline, serotonin and to a lesser extent dopamine have been linked with manic symptoms;
  - evidence in support of the monoamine theory:
    - cocaine increases levels of noradrenaline and adrenaline in the brain and can lead to manic symptoms,
    - tricyclic antidepressants (TCAs) in excess or used in bipolar disorder can induce hypomanic or manic episodes,
    - the use of the drug L-dopa in Parkinson's disease to increase dopamine levels can lead to manic symptoms;
  - the neurotransmitter glutamate has been linked with manic symptoms.
- Hormonal abnormalities:
  - decreased levels of growth hormone (GH) have been recorded in patients with mania (secondary to increased levels of the inhibitory hormone somatostatin);
  - increased levels of thyroid hormone (T_4) are known to cause manic symptoms (i.e. in hyperthyroidism).
- Biological factors:
  - sleep deprivation;
  - **kindling hypothesis**: the persistence of neuronal damage leads to recurrence of mania without precipitating factors. This is known as

kindling and subsequent manic episodes become more autonomous and frequent.
- Psychosocial factors:
  - significant life events and severe stressors can precipitate the onset of hypomania or mania.
- Cyclothymic personality disorder is linked with mania.

CLINICAL FEATURES

The symptoms of mania are displayed in Fig. 7.1.

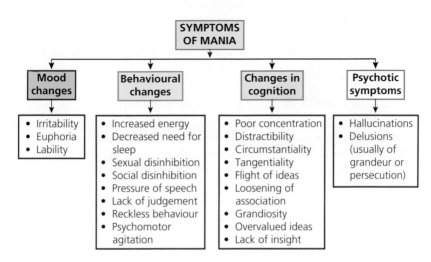

Fig. 7.1 **Symptoms of mania.**

- The ICD-10 specifies three degrees of severity for a single manic episode depending on the symptoms and degree of functional impairment (see Table 7.1).

MICRO-reference
http://apps.who.int/classifications/icd10/browse/2010/en

MICRO-facts
Remember that it is **impossible** for a patient to have a visual hallucination that talks to them as the two areas of the brain that this would involve are not able to communicate in such a way to facilitate this.

Table 7.1 Classification of manic episodes.

	HYPOMANIA	MANIA WITHOUT PSYCHOTIC SYMPTOMS	MANIA WITH PSYCHOTIC SYMPTOMS
Duration	Several days	More than 1 week	More than 1 week
Diagnostic guidelines	Typical but less severe manic symptoms Considerable but incomplete disruption to everyday life	Typical manic symptoms especially grandiosity, pressure of speech, excessive optimism and decreased need for sleep Complete disruption to work or social activity	Typical manic symptoms Delusions and/or hallucinations present Complete disruption to work or social activity
Other information	Often occurs immediately preceding or following onset of recovery from a manic episode	Patients may have perceptual disturbances such as preoccupation with textures or vivid colours	Includes manic stupor Important to determine if delusions or hallucinations are mood congruent or incongruent

INVESTIGATIONS

- As for most disorders in psychiatry the diagnosis for manic episode is clinical so investigations are aimed at ruling out other differential diagnoses (see Differential diagnosis below).
- Bloods:
  - full blood count (FBC);
  - urea and electrolytes (U&E);
  - liver function tests (LFTs);
  - thyroid function tests (TFTs);
  - serum calcium and parathyroid hormone (PTH);
  - vitamin B_{12} and folate;
  - human immunodeficiency virus (HIV) screen;
  - syphilis screen.
- Urine drug screen.
- Electroencephalogram (EEG).
- Computed tomography (CT) of head.

- It is important to get a **collateral history** from a family member, general practitioner (GP) or close friend.

DIFFERENTIAL DIAGNOSIS

- Neurological disease: multiple sclerosis, Huntington's disease, brain tumours, temporal lobe epilepsy.
- Infectious disease: HIV, acquired immune deficiency syndrome (AIDS), syphilis.
- Endocrinopathies: Cushing's syndrome, hyperthyroidism, parathyroid dysfunction.
- Vitamin deficiencies: vitamin B_{12}, folate, niacin.
- Others: renal failure, systemic lupus erythematosus (SLE).
- Substance use/abuse: cocaine, amphetamines, L-dopa, corticosteroids, antidepressants, anticholinergics, antiviral drugs, cimetidine.
- Other psychiatric disorders: schizophrenia, schizoaffective disorder, delirium, dementia, personality disorders, bipolar affective disorder, hypomania/mania/mixed affective episode, cyclothymia.

MANAGEMENT

- Acute episode:
    - hospitalization may be necessary if posing risk to self (e.g. from self-harm, reckless behaviour, neglect or exhaustion) or others (e.g. aggressive behaviours);
    - detention under the Mental Health Act may be appropriate;
    - pharmacological therapy if not already on anti-manic treatments:
        - an atypical antipsychotic licensed to treat mania (i.e. aripiprazole, olanzapine, risperidone or quetiapine),
        - a typical antipsychotic (e.g. haloperidol),
        - if inadequate response to antipsychotic add lithium or valproate,
        - base choice of second drug on discussion of side-effect profile with patient (if possible/appropriate),
        - avoid the use of lithium and valproate in women of childbearing age (severely teratogenic),

---

MICRO-facts

Lithium use in pregnancy causes Ebstein's anomaly while use of valproate causes neural tube defects.

        - other possible treatments include carbamazepine, lamotrigine and topiramate,
        - benzodiazepine use (e.g. lorazepam) can be very useful for agitation;

Mental health disorders

- patient currently on anti-manic treatment:
  - check compliance,
  - check plasma levels of drugs.
- Mania prophylaxis: see Management in the section Bipolar affective disorder below.
- Other therapies:
  - electroconvulsive therapy (ECT) can be useful if severe symptoms;
  - only use ECT if rapid and short-term improvement desired;
  - important to reduce or stop benzodiazepine before ECT commences;
  - psychological therapy is not very effective in mania.

PROGNOSIS

- Episodes typically last 2 weeks to 4 months.
- > 90% of patients will go on to have a further affective episode at which point the diagnosis is changed to **bipolar affective disorder** (see section on Bipolar affective disorder).

7.2 DEPRESSIVE EPISODE

EPIDEMIOLOGY

MICRO-case

Ms Z is a 36-year-old recently divorced mother of two who comes to see you as her GP because she has been feeling 'low' for the past 3 months. She tells you that since her divorce was finalized 2 years ago she has felt as if she doesn't have a purpose anymore as she is struggling to find a job having given up work to look after her children, now aged 6 and 8 years. She also says that she no longer finds enjoyment in painting or playing the piano – pastimes that she used to spend most of her spare time doing. During the consultation she is quite tearful as she says that she has considered going to the chemists and buying a few packs of paracetamol to 'end it all'. She admits that these thoughts then make her feel immensely guilty and she feels as if she is an unfit mother. She denies hearing voices, but on mentioning to her that she looks tired and thin she says that she wakes up at 4 a.m. most days and has lost over a stone in the past 6 weeks.

Learning point

- Depressive episodes can have both physical and psychological manifestations.

- Point prevalence: 2–5%.
- Mean age of onset: 27 years.
- Male to female ratio: 1:2.

AETIOLOGY

- Genetic factors:
  - family studies:
    - 40–70% chance of having a depressive episode if a first-degree family member has had one,
    - increased risk of having a depressive episode if family members suffer from anxiety disorders, alcohol dependence or other affective disorders;
  - twin studies:
    - 46–50% concordance in monozygotic twins,
    - 20% concordance in dizygotic twins;
  - adoption studies:
    - research has shown twofold greater risk if a biological parent suffers from depressive episodes.
- Neurotransmitter abnormalities:
  - monoamine theory: decreased levels of noradrenaline, serotonin and to a lesser extent dopamine have been linked with depressive symptoms;
  - evidence in support of the monoamine theory:
    - antidepressants increase levels of these neurotransmitters in the central nervous system (CNS),
    - many patients with Parkinson's disease (decreased basal ganglia dopaminergic activity) exhibit depressive symptoms;
  - decreased levels of gamma-aminobutyric acid (GABA) have been implicated in depressive disease;
  - some antidepressants upregulate GABA receptors;
  - acetylcholine has also been implicated since acetylcholine agonists can induce depressive symptoms of anergia, lethargy and psychomotor retardation.

> **MICRO-print**
> Although the monoamine theory is the most widely accepted explanation for the aetiology of depression, it is not fully understood. For example, drugs (e.g. cocaine) that temporarily increase the levels of these neurotransmitters within the brain are not effective as treatment for depression. It is likely, therefore, that correction of the depletion in these neurotransmitters needs to span a longer period of time to redress intracellular imbalances.

- Hormonal abnormalities:
  - increased levels of GH have been recorded in patients with depression (secondary to decreased levels of the inhibitory hormone somatostatin);

Mental health disorders

- decreased levels of T_4 are known to cause depressive symptoms (i.e. in hypothyroidism);
- increased levels of cortisol are found in some individuals with depression. Non-suppression in dexamethasone suppression test (DST) is greatest in people with severe depression and reversed with antidepressant treatment. Non-suppression of DST is a result of increased hypothalamic corticotrophin releasing factor (CRF) release.
- Psychosocial factors:
  - adverse life events often precede the onset of the first episode but not necessarily subsequent episodes, suggesting that a single depressive episode may lead to lasting changes in the brain;
  - marital status:
    - greater risk in divorced individuals over married ones (married < divorced < single),
    - three times greater risk in unemployed individuals;
  - childhood risk factors:
    - sexual abuse,
    - parental alcoholism,
    - loss of parent,
    - failure to form appropriate attachment in early life.
- Concurrent medical illness, especially post-myocardial infarction, diabetes mellitus, cancer and neurological disease (e.g. multiple sclerosis).

MICRO-facts

Brown and Harris' *Social origins of depression* (1978)
They found the following risk factors for the development of depression in women:

- 3 or more children at home under the age of 14;
- lack of employment;
- lack of confiding relationship.

MICRO-reference
Brown GW, Harris T. *Social origins of depression: a study of psychiatric disorder in women.* London: Tavistock Publications Limited, 1978

- Concurrent psychiatric disorders:
  - the following often coexist with depression/predispose to depressive illness:
    - obsessive–compulsive disorder (OCD),
    - alcohol abuse or dependence,
    - panic disorder,

- social anxiety disorder,
- histrionic personality disorder,
- anankastic personality disorder,
- borderline personality disorder.

MICRO-print

Sleep cycle changes in depression:

- decreased slow wave sleep (due to decreased GH secretion);
- increased rapid eye movement (REM) sleep with decreased intervals between REM sleep.

Manifestations of sleep cycle changes:

- decreased total sleep time;
- increased nocturnal awakenings;
- early morning awakening (terminal insomnia).

CLINICAL FEATURES

- Three key features:
  - depressed mood:
    - not influenced by circumstance,
    - varies little from day to day, but may show diurnal variation;
  - anhedonia:
    - lack of enjoyment or interest in activities that were formerly pleasurable to the individual;
  - anergia:
    - can present either as fatigue or lack of motivation,
    - leads to diminished activity.
- Other symptoms:
  - decreased concentration and attention (i.e. easily distracted);
  - poor self-esteem and loss of confidence;
  - feelings of guilt, often out of proportion to original offence;
  - bleak and pessimistic views of the future;
  - ideas of self-harm and suicide (see Chapter 15 Psychiatric emergencies, Suicide and Self-harm);
  - diminished appetite;
  - disturbed sleep, especially early morning wakening.
- For diagnosis the depressive symptoms need to have been present for the majority of the time over the past 2 weeks.
- A person is said to be suffering from atypical depression if they are exhibiting the following symptoms:
  - hypersomnia,
  - over-eating.

- The ICD-10 categorizes depressive episodes into the following groups depending on severity of symptoms (Fig. 7.2):
  - mild depressive episode;
  - moderate depressive episode;
  - severe depressive episode without psychotic symptoms;
  - severe depressive episode with psychotic symptoms.

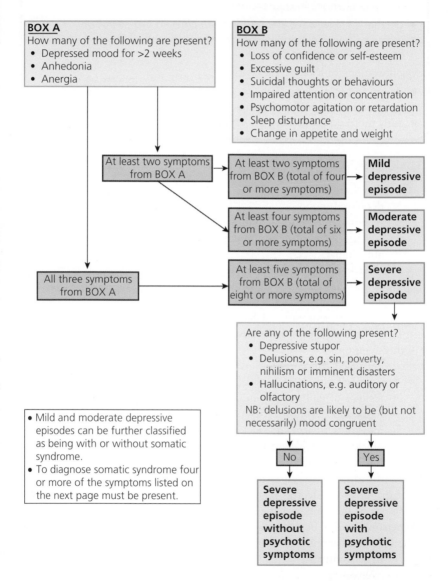

Fig. 7.2 Classification of depressive episodes.

- Melancholic depression is stated by the DSM-IV-TR but not the ICD-10. The features include:
  - loss of pleasure in all activities;
  - lack of reactivity to usually pleasurable stimuli;
  - distinct quality of depressed mood;
  - depression regularly worse in the morning;
  - early morning awakening;
  - marked psychomotor retardation;
  - significant anorexia and weight loss;
  - excessive or inappropriate guilt.

MICRO-reference

American Psychiatric Association. *Diagnostic and statistical manual of mental disorders*, 4th edn (text revision). Washington, DC: American Psychiatric Association, 2000.

- Somatic syndrome:
  - weight loss of more than 5% in the past month;
  - loss of libido;
  - terminal insomnia or early morning wakening (waking usually more than 2 hours before the usual time);
  - loss of emotional reactivity to events or activities that normally produce emotional responses;
  - symptoms worse in the morning;
  - anhedonia;
  - psychomotor retardation or agitation;
  - loss of appetite.

MICRO-facts

Use the following mnemonic to help you remember the symptoms in the somatic syndrome:

When (weight loss)

Leftover (loss of libido)

Takeaway is (terminal insomnia)

Eaten in the (loss of emotional reactivity)

Morning (worse symptoms in the morning)

Awful (anhedonia)

Pains (psychomotor retardation/agitation)

Arise (appetite loss)

Mental health disorders

- Signs of depression:
  - self-neglect (e.g. hair, clothing, weight loss, poor personal hygeine);
  - poor eye contact;
  - sagging corners of mouth;
  - psychomotor retardation/agitation;
  - anxiety;
  - irritability;
  - slow speech;
  - latent interval before answering;
  - single word answers;
  - decreased inflection;
  - decreased volume of speech;
  - decreased pace of speech;
  - decreased cognition (pseudodementia).

INVESTIGATIONS

- As for manic episode the diagnosis is mostly clinical so investigations are aimed at ruling out other differential diagnoses.
- Bloods:
  - FBC;
  - U&E;
  - LFTs;
  - TFTs;
  - serum calcium and PTH;
  - vitamin B_{12} and folate;
  - HIV screen;
  - syphilis screen.
- Urine drug screen.
- CT of head.
- It is important to get a collateral history from a family member, GP or close friend.
- Two questions can be used to effectively screen for depression:
  - During the past month how often have you been bothered by feeling down, depressed or hopeless?
  - During the past month how often have you been bothered by having little interest or pleasure in doing things?
- The Patient Health Questionnaire (PHQ-9) is a tool used by GPs to determine how likely a person is to have depression:
  - it uses the DSM-IV criteria for depression, not the ICD-10;
  - it consists of nine questions;
  - it can also be used to monitor an individual's response to treatment in primary care.

> **MICRO-reference**
> PHQ-9 copyrights are held by Pfizer Inc. and as such a sample of the tool is not reproduced here. It may be accessed at: http://www.phqscreeners.com/overview.aspx?Screener=02_PHQ-9

- It is imperative to do a full suicide risk assessment on any patient presenting with depressive symptoms (see Chapter 15 Psychiatric emergencies, Suicide).

DIFFERENTIAL DIAGNOSIS

Differential diagnoses for depressive episodes are given in Table 7.2.

Table 7.2 Differential diagnoses for depressive episodes.

Neurological disease	MS, Parkinson's disease, Huntington's disease, stroke, head injury, brain tumour, neurosyphilis, HIV/AIDS, Wernicke's encephalopathy
Endocrine and metabolic disease	Hypothyroidism, parathyroid dysfunction, hypoglycaemia, Cushing's disease, Addison's disease, hypopituitarism, prolactinoma
Psychiatric illnesses	Depressive episode, recurrent depressive disorder, bipolar affective disorder, dysthymia, cyclothymia, dementia, substance abuse (especially alcoholism), schizoaffective disorder, eating disorders, personality disorders, anxiety disorders
Others	Menstrual disorders, insomnia, chronic fatigue syndrome, obstructive sleep apnoea, SLE, acute intermittent porphyria, renal failure, malignancy, rheumatoid arthritis, vitamin deficiencies
Prescribed drugs	Corticosteroids, combined oral contraceptive pill, opiates, antipsychotics, L-dopa, beta-blockers, phenytoin, benzodiazepines, carbamezapine

AIDS, acquired immune deficiency syndrome; HIV, human immunodeficiency virus; MS, multiple sclerosis; SLE, systemic lupus erythematosus.

MANAGEMENT

- Stop any medications that may be contributing to the mood disturbance.
- Offer sleep hygiene advice (see Chapter 9 Behavioural syndromes associated with physiological disturbance, Sleep disorders).
- Hospitalization may be appropriate if the individual poses severe threat to self or others through aggression, neglect, self-harm or suicide.

Mental health disorders

- Pharmacological therapy:
  - antidepressants (see Chapter 13 Pharmacotherapy, Antidepressants):
    - do not use for mild or sub-threshold depressive symptoms lasting less than 2 years,
    - need to inform patient that it can take 4–6 weeks for maximal response to drug;
  - choosing antidepressants:
    - a thorough discussion of potential side-effects needs to be undertaken,
    - first line – selective serotonin re-uptake inhibitors (SSRIs);
  - augmenting antidepressants:
    - if inadequate response to single drug treatment, other agents such as lithium, an antipsychotic (such as aripiprazole, olanzapine, quetiapine or risperidone) or other antidepressants (such as mirtazapine) can be added (see Chapter 13 Pharmacotherapy, Antipsychotics and Mood stabilizers),
    - if the individual is suffering from psychotic symptoms add one of the above-mentioned antipsychotics;
  - antidepressants are normally continued for 6 months to 2 years depending on the individual's response and severity of the episode.
- Psychological therapy:
  - should be offered to all patients with depressive symptoms;
  - mild to moderate depression:
    - 3–4 months of low-intensity intervention:
      - ○ computerized cognitive behavioural therapy (CCBT),
      - ○ group physical activity session,
      - ○ group cognitive behavioural therapy (CBT) if the above are inappropriate;
  - severe depression or if poor treatment response:
    - 3–4 months of high-intensity intervention:
      - ○ CBT,
      - ○ interpersonal therapy (IPT),
      - ○ behavioural couples therapy,
      - ○ behavioural activation.

MICRO-facts

Behavioural couples therapy is useful if the partner is thought to either be contributing to the depressive illness or has a positive role in the recovery process.

- Electroconvulsive therapy:
  - highly effective in severe life-threatening depression, e.g. imminent suicide risk;
  - can be useful if all other treatments have failed;
  - can be used if patient is refusing to eat or drink;
  - do not routinely use for moderate depression unless all other treatment options have failed;
  - fully informed consent must be gained and the patient informed about side-effects of general anaesthetic as well as potential side-effects of the treatment such as cognitive impairment.

PROGNOSIS

- About 60% of patients will have a further episode (at which point the diagnosis is changed to recurrent depressive disorder).
- If untreated, a mild/moderate episode will usually last for 4–30 days.
- If untreated, a severe episode will last, on average, 6 months.

7.3 RECURRENT DEPRESSIVE DISORDER

EPIDEMIOLOGY

- Prevalence: similar to depressive episode (see the section on Depressive episode, above).
- Mean age of onset: fifth decade.
- Male to female ratio: 1:2.

AETIOLOGY

- As for depressive episode (see the section on Depressive episode, above).
- Episodes are often precipitated by stressful life events.

CLINICAL FEATURES

- Recurrent episodes of depressed mood.
- Similar classification (i.e. mild/moderate/severe and with or without somatic syndrome) as for depressive episode (see the section on Depressive episode, above).
- Episodes should last for at least 2 weeks and usually last 3–12 months.
- There should be several months of remission between episodes.
- Recurrent depressive episode currently in remission:
  - used to describe the current state of a patient in whom at least two previous depressive episodes have been diagnosed but who does not currently suffer from depressive symptoms;

Mental health disorders

- can be used to describe a patient receiving treatment for a previous depressive episode and whose symptoms are currently well controlled.

INVESTIGATIONS, DIFFERENTIAL DIAGNOSIS AND MANAGEMENT

- As for depressive episode (see the section on Depressive episode, above).

PROGNOSIS

Prognostic factors in recurrent depressive disorder are outlined in Table 7.3.
- Median duration of episodes is 6 months.
- Usually complete recovery between episodes.
- Persistent depressive symptoms may occur in old age.
- Risk of relapse increases with increasing number of depressive episodes.
- Twenty times greater risk of suicide compared with the general population.
- A 60–70% remission rate with antidepressant therapy.
- Risk factors for recurrence:
    - residual symptoms such as low mood, sleep disturbance, anxiety or decreased libido.

Table 7.3 Prognostic factors in recurrent depressive disorder.

FACTORS ASSOCIATED WITH GOOD PROGNOSIS	FACTORS ASSOCIATED WITH POOR PROGNOSIS
Acute onset	Insidious onset
Endogenous depression	Neurotic depression
Early age of onset	Residual symptoms
	Elderly age
	Low self-confidence
	Comorbid medical or psychiatric illness
	Lack of social support

MICRO-reference

National Institute for Health and Clinical Excellence. *Depression in adults. CG90.* London: National Institute for Health and Clinical Excellence, 2009.

7.4 BIPOLAR AFFECTIVE DISORDER

EPIDEMIOLOGY

- Prevalence: 0.3–1.5%.
- Prevalence of bipolar I: 0.2–4%.
- Prevalence of bipolar II: 0.3–4.8%.
- Mean age of onset: 20 years.
- Male to female ratio: 1:1.

> **MICRO-facts**
>
> **DSM-IV classification**
>
> **Bipolar I:** major depression has occurred alongside at least one episode of mania.
>
> **Bipolar II:** major depression has occurred alongside hypomania (but **not** mania) at least once.

- Women tend to have more depressive episodes.
- Men tend to have more manic episodes.
- Women have a higher rate of rapid cycling bipolar affective disorder (BAD) (≥4 episodes in a year).

AETIOLOGY

- As for manic episode and depressive episode (see the sections on Manic episode and Depressive episode above).

> **MICRO-facts**
>
> Severe depression and mania are often seen as two ends of a spectrum between which a patient with bipolar affective disorder will alternate. This is reflected in the current theories regarding aetiology of the mood disorders.

- Genetic factors:
  - there is a proposed shared genetic link between BAD, schizophrenia and schizoaffective disorder.
  - family studies:
    - seven times more likely to develop BAD if a first-degree relative has it;
  - twin studies:
    - 65–75% concordance rate in monozygotic twins,
    - 14% concordance rate in dizygotic twins;

Mental health disorders

- adoption studies:
  - three times greater risk of developing BAD than the general population if a biological parent suffers from it.

MICRO-print

A study by Ferreira et al. (2008) compiling data from their findings and three other studies showed that two gene mutations coding for ion channels in the central nervous system are more frequently seen in patients with BAD. This suggests the possibility of a channelopathy as an aetiological factor. The genes are ANK3 (ankyrin G) on chromosome 10q21 and CACNA1C (alpha 1C subunit of L-type voltage-gated calcium channel) on chromosome 12p13.

MICRO-reference

Ferreira MAR, O'Donovan MC, Meng YA, Jones IR, Ruderfer DM, Jones L et al. Collaborative genome wide association analysis supports a role for ANK3 and CACNA1C in bipolar disorder. Nat Genet 2008; **40**:1056–8.

- Psychosocial factors:
  - significant life events often precede the onset of the first episode;
  - pregnancy can trigger an episode in a woman with pre-existing BAD;
  - cyclothymic personality disorder can predispose to BAD.

CLINICAL FEATURES

- Repeated (≥ 2) episodes of significant mood and activity disturbance.
- Episodes are sometimes hypomanic/manic and sometimes depressed.
- Episodes must last for ≥ 2 weeks.

MICRO-facts

People who experience repeated episodes of purely hypomanic or manic symptoms, in the absence of illicit drug use, are diagnosed as having BAD. 'Recurrent manic disorder' is not a recognized diagnosis.

- ICD-10 classification:
  - BAD, current episode hypomanic;
  - BAD, current episode manic without psychotic symptoms;
  - BAD, current episode manic with psychotic symptoms;
  - BAD, current episode mild/moderate depression;
  - BAD, current episode severe depression without psychotic symptoms;

- BAD, current episode severe depression with psychotic symptoms;
- BAD, current episode mixed;
- BAD, currently in remission.
- For details of criteria see sections on Manic episode and Depressive episode above.
- You can further classify the depressive episodes as with or without somatic syndrome.

MICRO-facts

Mixed affective episode:

- Patient exhibits mixed affective symptoms (e.g. elated mood with anergia and loss of libido).
- Both types of symptoms must be present for the greater part of the current episode.
- Symptoms can rapidly alternate.

- Rapid cycling:
  - ≥ 4 episodes of mood disturbance in a year.

INVESTIGATIONS AND DIFFERENTIAL DIAGNOSIS

- As for manic episode and depressive episode (see relevant topics in the sections on Manic episode and Depressive episode above).

MANAGEMENT

- Hospitalization:
  - if symptoms rapidly worsening and unmanageable in the community and posing significant risk to self and/or others (e.g. through reckless behaviour, self-neglect or self-harming);
  - detention under the Mental Health Act may be appropriate.
- Manic episodes:
  - for acute treatment see section on Manic episode;
  - if a patient is already on a mood stabilizer check dose and consider adding an antipsychotic;
  - prophylaxis:
    - use of long-term mood stabilizers is very effective at preventing relapses,
    - drugs used are lithium, olanzapine and semisodium valproate,
    - base choice of drug on patient preference after full discussion of potential side-effects,
    - avoid the use of lithium and semisodium valproate in women of childbearing age as they are severely teratogenic,

- if response is unsatisfactory switch to another drug or add a second agent (e.g. lithium plus valproate),
- continue treatment for at least 2 years after an episode of BAD or up to 5 years if there is significant risk of relapse.

MICRO-facts

Think about contraception for all women of childbearing age as sexual disinhibition is often seen in mania.

- Depressive episodes:
  - beware using antidepressants as can provoke hypomanic or manic symptoms;
  - if absolutely necessary to give an antidepressant ALWAYS prescribe a mood stabilizer as well;
  - first line – SSRIs (e.g. fluoxetine);
  - do not routinely use lamotrigine as a single first-line treatment, although it is useful in rapid-cycling BAD;
  - the atypical agent quetiapine has been shown to be highly effective in BAD;
  - mild symptoms:
    - review patient in 1–2 weeks,
    - do not give antidepressant;
  - moderate symptoms and unsatisfactory response to drugs:
    - consider psychotherapy as for depressive episode;
  - stop antidepressant therapy after 8 weeks of depressive symptom resolution, but continue mood stabilizer as detailed above under manic episode prophylaxis.
- Mixed affective episodes:
  - do not start antidepressant therapy;
  - stabilize symptoms on mood stabilizers.
- Psychological therapy:
  - psychotherapy is not as useful for BAD as it is for depression;
  - can be useful if severe depressive symptoms not responding to pharmacological therapy (use CBT);
  - family intervention can be useful.

PROGNOSIS

Prognostic factors in bipolar affective disorder are outlined in Table 7.4.
- Manic episodes typically begin abruptly and last for 2 weeks to 4 months.
- Depressive episodes last, on average, 6 months.
- Remission time is variable and decreases with increasing age.

- 60–70% remission rate with lithium therapy.
- 15–19% suicide risk (more common in depressive episodes).
- Worse prognosis than for depression.

Table 7.4 Prognostic factors in bipolar affective disorder.

FACTORS ASSOCIATED WITH GOOD PROGNOSIS	FACTORS ASSOCIATED WITH POOR PROGNOSIS
Short duration of manic episode	Poor employment history
Later age of onset	Alcohol abuse
Few or no suicidal thoughts	Depressive symptoms between episodes
Few psychotic symptoms	Psychotic features
Few comorbid physical problems	Male sex
Good response to treatment	Poor response to treatment
Good treatment compliance	Poor treatment compliance

MICRO-reference

National Institute for Health and Clinical Excellence. *Bipolar disorder. CG38.* London: National Institute for Health and Clinical Excellence, 2006.

7.5 OTHER AFFECTIVE DISORDERS

DYSTHYMIA

- Epidemiology:
    - prevalence: 6%;
    - age of onset: childhood/adolescence/early adulthood;
    - male to female ratio: 1:2.
- Aetiology:
    - links to decreased serotonin and noradrenaline;
    - patients exhibit decreased REM sleep latency as for depressive episodes;
    - links with borderline personality disorder and anxiety disorders.
- Clinical features:
    - chronically depressed mood not satisfying criteria for recurrent depressive disorder in terms of severity or duration;
    - variable periods of wellness;
    - symptoms must be present for ≥2 years;

- common symptoms:
  - fatigue,
  - poor appetite,
  - sleep disturbance,
  - low self-esteem,
  - decreased concentration,
  - difficulty making decisions.
- Investigations and differential diagnosis:
  - as for depressive episode (see section on Depressive episode above);
  - clinical diagnosis;
  - PHQ-9 is effective to distinguish from recurrent depressive disorder.
- Management:
  - good response rate to SSRIs (e.g. fluoxetine);
  - similar dose and regime of antidepressants as for depressive episode;
  - CBT and IPT can be very effective.
- Prognosis:
  - chronic course;
  - 30–70% response rate to antidepressants;
  - can coexist with depressive episodes (so called 'double depression');
  - poorer prognosis if comorbid personality disorders or anxiety disorders.

CYCLOTHYMIA

MICRO-facts

Cyclothymia is often underdiagnosed as many patients enjoy the feelings of mild elation and therefore do not seek medical attention. Patients are more likely to seek medical attention in episodes of mild depression.

- Epidemiology:
  - prevalence: 0.5–1%;
  - age of onset: early adulthood;
  - male to female ratio: 1:2.
- Aetiology:
  - up to one-third of patients will have relatives with BAD.
- Clinical features:
  - persistent mood instability with numerous periods of mild elation and depression;
  - variable periods of wellness;
  - periods of mood disturbance are not severe enough to fulfil criteria for manic or depressive episodes;
  - periods of mood disturbance are unrelated to life events.

- Management:
  - as for BAD in its mildest form (see the section on Recurrent depressive disorder above);
  - do not use antidepressants as these can induce hypomanic or manic symptoms;
  - if the use of drugs needs to be considered use a mood stabilizer (e.g. lithium);
  - psychoeducation:
    - used for patient understanding,
    - helps patient develop better coping techniques.
- Prognosis:
  - chronic course persisting throughout adult life;
  - periods of stability may be present for months at a time.

SEASONAL AFFECTIVE DISORDER

- Definition:
  - atypical depressive symptoms seen in relation to a particular time of the year.
- Epidemiology:
  - prevalence: 2%;
  - average age of onset: 30 years;
  - male to female ratio: 1:5.
- Aetiology:
  - increased melatonin synthesis during the winter months leading to typical symptoms (e.g. fatigue);
  - decreased serotonin availability leads to depressive symptoms;
  - increased risk in individuals with a first-degree relative with seasonal affective disorder (SAD).
- Clinical features:
  - usually occurs from September to April;
  - symptoms are worse in January and February;
  - typical symptoms:
    - low mood,
    - low self-esteem,
    - hypersomnia,
    - fatigue,
    - increased appetite,
    - weight gain,
    - decreased social functioning,
    - anhedonia,
    - poor concentration,
    - loss of libido;

> **MICRO-facts**
>
> It is important to establish that depressive symptoms are not caused by any exogenous factor that occurs during the winter (e.g. unemployment during the winter months).

- symptoms must be present for ≥ 2 years.
- Management:
  - light therapy:
    - simulates sunlight throughout the winter months,
    - used on waking,
    - antidepressant effect seen within 2–5 days (but can be much longer),
    - unavailable on the National Health Service (NHS),
    - ~65% response rate;
  - pharmacological therapy:
    - SSRIs can be effective (e.g. fluoxetine),
    - propranolol to suppress melatonin secretion;
  - psychological therapy:
    - CBT can be a useful adjuvant therapy.

BEREAVEMENT

- **Phase I: shock and protest** includes numbness, disbelief and acute dysphoria.
- **Phase II: preoccupation** includes yearning, searching and anger.
- **Phase III: disorganization** includes despair and acceptance of loss.
- **Phase IV: resolution**.
- A person may develop depressive episode after bereavement. The following features suggest of depressive episode:
  - guilt, suicidal thoughts and hallucinations not related to the deceased;
  - feelings of worthlessness;
  - psychomotor retardation;
  - prolonged and marked functional impairment.

PATHOLOGICAL GRIEF

- Inhibited grief: absence of expected grief symptoms at any stage.
- Delayed grief: avoidance of painful symptoms within 2 weeks of loss.
- Chronic grief: continued significant grief-related symptoms 6 months after loss.

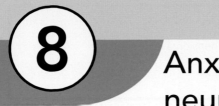

Anxiety and neuroses

8.1 GENERALIZED ANXIETY DISORDER

EPIDEMIOLOGY

- Prevalence: 5%.
- Male to female ratio: male > female.
- Commonest in early adulthood.
- Associated with other mood disorders.

AETIOLOGY

- Genetic factors:
  - heritability is around 30%;
  - increased risk in first-degree relatives thought to result from genetic factors.
- Personality:
  - associated with neuroticism (personality trait);
  - associated with anxious-avoidant personality disorder (see Chapter 10 Disorders of adult personality, Classification).
- Life events:
  - triggered by stressful life events;
  - more prevalent in those who have been involved in a traumatic event (e.g. a bomb attack or natural disaster).
- Home environment:
  - separation in childhood;
  - anxious mother;
  - emotional trauma during childhood.

CLINICAL FEATURES

MICRO-facts

Diagnostic criteria (based on ICD-10):

- Must have symptoms most days for several weeks/months.

continued...

continued...

- Symptoms involve:
  - free-floating anxiety/apprehension;
  - motor tension;
  - autonomic over-activity.

MICRO-reference
http://apps.who.int/classifications/icd10/browse/2010/en

- Psychological symptoms:
  - feeling of threat/foreboding (not specific);
  - difficulty concentrating;
  - feeling on edge, tense and unable to relax;
  - irritability;
  - early insomnia;
  - fear of loss (not specific).
- Motor tension:
  - tension headache;
  - restlessness;
  - muscular tension.
- Autonomic symptoms:
  - sweating;
  - flushing;
  - frequent urination;
  - tachycardia;
  - breathlessness;
  - dry mouth;
  - dizziness.

SCREENING QUESTIONS

- Do you feel worried a lot (how many days in last month)?
- Do you worry about anything in particular (e.g. finances)?
- What sort of symptoms do you get when you feel worried (e.g. tachycardia)?
- Has it interfered with your ability to perform your usual activities/work?
- Do symptoms increase with stimulants such as caffeine?
- Ask about medications used (as could be causing symptoms).
- Screen for depression (see Chapter 7 Affective disorders, Depressive episode).

INVESTIGATIONS

- Thyroid function tests (TFTs): to exclude thyrotoxicosis as cause of anxiety.
- Blood glucose: to exclude hypoglycaemia as cause of anxiety.

- Electrocardiogram (ECG) and cardiac echocardiography: to exclude atrial fibrillation and other cardiac problems as causing anxiety.
- Lung function tests: to exclude hyperventilation as cause of anxiety.
- Urine toxicology screen: to exclude stimulant use as cause of anxiety.

MANAGEMENT

- Acute or emergency use:
  - benzodiazepines can be used in crises, but should not be used for longer than 2–4 weeks.
- Long term:
  - education:
    - information leaflets and self-monitoring;
  - psychological therapy:
    - low-intensity interventions:
      - self-help guides,
      - computerized cognitive behavioural therapy (CCBT),
      - support groups;
    - high-intensity interventions:
      - cognitive behavioural therapy (CBT): effective for longest; delivered in weekly sessions for 16–20 hours in total;
  - pharmacological therapy:
    - selective serotonin re-uptake inhibitors (SSRIs) (e.g. paroxetine) licensed for generalized anxiety disorder (GAD),
    - mirtazapine, venlafaxine, pregabalin and duloxetine all have a good evidence base,
    - buspirone (anxiolytic),
    - beta-blocker (e.g. propranolol) for somatic symptoms.

PROGNOSIS

- In most patients this is a chronic condition which may improve with CBT but it may reoccur with future life events and stresses.
- Poor prognostic factors include severe anxiety symptoms, frequent syncope, derealization and suicide attempts.

8.2 MIXED ANXIETY AND DEPRESSION

- Patients presenting with anxiety will often also suffer from depression.
- Important to screen for both.
- Diagnosis used when both conditions are present but neither is severe enough to justify a diagnosis on its own.
- Treat most prominent symptoms as appropriate from depression and anxiety management.

Mental health disorders

8.3 PANIC DISORDER

EPIDEMIOLOGY

- Prevalence: 1%.
- Male to female ratio: 1:2.
- Commonly develops in twenties.

AETIOLOGY

- Genetic factors:
  - high risk of panic disorder in individuals with an affected first-degree relative (15–30%).
- Life events:
  - people who have experienced a stressful life event are at high risk of panic disorder in the following year.
- Neurotransmitter abnormalities:
  - abnormal activity of presynaptic alpha$_2$-adrenoreceptors and increase in adrenergic activities;
  - yohimbine (a supplement) has high affinity for the alpha$_2$-adrenergic receptors and it may induce panic attacks;
  - 5-hydroxytryptamine (5-HT; subsensitivity of $5HT_{1A}$ receptors and exaggerated post-synaptic receptor response) and benzodiazepine receptors have also been suggested as important.

CLINICAL FEATURES

> ## MICRO-facts
>
> Common features of a panic attack:
> - sudden onset of fear and autonomic symptoms;
> - palpitations;
> - chest pain;
> - dizziness;
> - choking sensation;
> - depersonalization/derealization (feel they or the situation are not real).
>
> These can then lead to a fear of dying.

- Several severe attacks occur within a period of a month.
- Unrelated to a specific situation/phobia.
- Free of anxiety symptoms between attacks (although there may be fear of having another attack).
- Length and frequency of attacks are variable.

SCREENING QUESTIONS

- Can you describe the symptoms to me?
- How do you feel between the attacks?
- Is there anything that triggers the attacks?
- Screen for anxiety (see the section on Generalized anxiety disorder above), phobias (see the section on Specific phobia) and depression (see Chapter 7 Affective disorders, Depressive episode).
- Screen for substance abuse (see Chapter 5 Substance misuse, Assessment of substance misuse).
- Hyperventilation syndrome and panic disorder share many common features and may also occur together (Table 8.1).
- It is important to ask about features of both.

Table 8.1 Comparison of panic disorder and hyperventilation syndrome.

	PANIC DISORDER	HYPERVENTILATION SYNDROME
Aetiology	Biological and psychological causes are well defined	Caffeine, lactate and psychological stressors play a role
Features	Autonomic arousal, mental symptoms	High thoracic breathing and excessive use of accessory muscles leads to hyperinflated lungs
Metabolic disturbances	Few	Acute hypocalcaemia, hypokalaemia, respiratory alkalosis
Investigations	TFTs, ECG, 24-hour urine catecholamines	Rule out PE with d-dimer and CTPA
Management	Pharmacotherapy	Relaxation techniques and breathing exercises

CTPA, computed tomography pulmonary angiogram; ECG, electrocardiogram; PE, pulmonary embolism; TFTs, thyroid function tests.

INVESTIGATIONS

- TFTs: to exclude thyrotoxicosis as cause of symptoms.
- ECG: to exclude arrhythmias as cause of symptoms.
- 24-hour urine catecholamines (especially if hypertension coexists): to exclude phaeochromocytoma as cause of symptoms.

Mental health disorders

MANAGEMENT

- Self-help and monitoring in primary care:
  - exercise for good general health;
  - bibliotherapy;
  - support groups.
- Psychological therapy:
  - CBT:
    - effective for longest,
    - delivered in weekly sessions for 7–14 hours in total.
- Pharmacological therapy:
  - SSRI (e.g. citalopram) for 12 weeks with regular review;
  - second line use clomipramine (unlicensed);
  - other treatments include mirtazapine, valproate, venlafaxine and monoamine oxidase inhibitors (MAOIs);
  - benzodiazepines or antipsychotics should not be prescribed for panic disorder.

PROGNOSIS

- The course of the illness is variable between patients with some having long-term problems while others respond well to CBT.

8.4 SPECIFIC PHOBIA

EPIDEMIOLOGY

- Prevalence: ~10%.
- Most common type of anxiety disorder.
- Usually arises in childhood (ages 4–12 years).
- May persist into adult life.

AETIOLOGY

- Home environment:
  - can often be traced back to a traumatic episode in childhood (e.g. phobia of dogs after being bitten by a dog);
  - children may develop a phobia through observational learning of the reactions of others around them.
- Genetic factors:
  - higher risk of developing a phobia if a first-degree relative has that phobia.

CLINICAL FEATURES

- Symptoms highly specific to:
  - certain situations (e.g. flying, crowds);

- certain objects, including living things (e.g. spiders, needles);
- natural phenomena (e.g. thunderstorms).
- Symptoms of anxiety only in the presence of the specific phobia.
- Avoidance of all circumstances that may trigger symptoms and anticipatory anxiety.

SCREENING QUESTIONS

- Are you scared of any situations or objects?
- What happens when you encounter this situation/object?
- Do you get these symptoms at any other time?
- Do you go out of your way to avoid this situation?
- How does this affect your life?

MANAGEMENT

- Psychological therapy:
  - talking therapies are mainly used:
    - counselling to discuss anxieties and reasons behind fear,
    - CBT to change response to phobia;
  - exposure and desensitization:
    - the person is gradually exposed to their phobia over time so they feel less anxious.
- Pharmacological therapy:
  - medication can be used if unavoidable (e.g. in fear of flying);
  - benzodiazepines;
  - beta-blockers (e.g. propranolol).

PROGNOSIS

- With appropriate therapy prognosis is good; however, if left untreated phobias can worsen over time and become very debilitating.

8.5 AGORAPHOBIA

EPIDEMIOLOGY

- Prevalence: affects ∼4% women and 2% men in a year.
- Male to female ratio: 1:2.
- Usually develops in early adulthood (18–35 years).

CLINICAL FEATURES

- Fear of open spaces but also including:
  - crowded places;
  - being unable to make an immediate exit to a safe place (usually home).
- Can result in being unable to leave the house.

Mental health disorders

- Criteria:
  - phobia caused by anxiety not secondary to delusion or obsession;
  - anxiety occurs mainly in public places, crowds, travelling (especially alone);
  - avoidance of the situation that provokes anxiety.
- May exist with or without panic disorder (see the section on Panic disorder).
- May lead to depression, social phobia and obsessional thoughts.

SCREENING QUESTIONS

- Do you start to feel anxious in public places (or other situations as described in the section on Agoraphobia)?
- Do you avoid situations for fear of developing anxiety symptoms (for example, going shopping)?
- Is this avoidance starting to impact on your life?
- Do you only get symptoms of anxiety when away from home?
- Do you suffer from panic attacks in public places? (See the section on Panic disorder.)
- Also screen for general anxiety disorder and depression (see Chapter 7 Affective disorders, Depressive episode and the section on Generalized anxiety disorder above).

MANAGEMENT

- Psychological therapy:
  - CBT:
    - to tackle concerns; for example, hyperventilation or fear of losing control.
  - desensitization:
    - gradually introduces the patient to their phobia to try and decrease their response.
- Pharmacological therapy:
  - SSRI antidepressants are first line, best used in combination with psychological therapy.

PROGNOSIS

- Varies depending on response to treatment.
- Anxiety may remain.

8.6 SOCIAL PHOBIA

EPIDEMIOLOGY

- 1-year incidence rate: ~10%.
- Male to female ratio: 1:1.
- Often begins in adolescence.

AETIOLOGY

* Sometimes related back to one embarrassing event in the past.

CLINICAL FEATURES

> **MICRO-facts**
>
> Diagnostic criteria (based on ICD-10):
> * symptoms only caused by anxiety not by any other disorder;
> * anxiety restricted to **social situation** (general or specific);
> * situation is avoided whenever possible.

* Anxiety brought on by fear of social situations.
* May be general and in any social situation outside of family/close friends.
* May be specific (e.g. eating in public, giving presentations).
* Often linked to low confidence and self-esteem.
* May be caused by fear of criticism.
* If severe, may lead to social isolation and problems at work.

SCREENING QUESTIONS

* Do you worry about social situations when you are the focus of attention?
* Do you avoid social situations?
* Do you get anxiety symptoms in social situations?
* Have you ever have a panic attack because of a social situation?
* Is this affecting your personal or work life?
* Screen for GAD and depression (see Chapter 7 Affective disorders, Depressive episode and the section on Generalized anxiety disorder above).

MANAGEMENT

* Psychological therapy:
    * CBT;
    * exposure therapy.
* Pharmacological therapy:
    * beta-blockers:
        - may ease symptoms of anxiety and help in less severe forms;
    * antidepressants:
        - may help reduce symptoms of social phobia even if not depressed.

PROGNOSIS

* Varies depending on response to treatment.
* May be life-long if left untreated.

Mental health disorders

8.7 OBSESSIVE–COMPULSIVE DISORDER

EPIDEMIOLOGY

- 1-year incidence rate: 1–3%.
- Male to female ratio: 1:1.
- Can begin in childhood but often starts in adolescence or early 20s.

AETIOLOGY

- Genetic factors:
  - there is an increased prevalence in monozygotic twins and first-degree relatives;
  - heritability is 30%;
  - polymorphisms in serotonergic, dopaminergic and gamma-aminobutyric acid (GABA) receptor genes have all been implicated.
- Neuroanatomical and neurotransmitter abnormalities:
  - dysfunction of the cortico-striatal-thalamic-cortical circuitry is seen;
  - serotonin and dopamine are both believed to play a role in obsessive–compulsive disorder (OCD).
- Life events:
  - may be triggered by a traumatic life event in those predisposed to the condition.
- Personality:
  - related to the anankastic personality type (see Chapter 10 Disorders of adult personality, Classification).

CLINICAL FEATURES

MICRO-facts

Obsession: an unwanted repetitive thought, image or urge that enters a person's mind.

Compulsion: a repetitive behaviour that a person feels they have to perform. Either physical (e.g. turning lights on and off) or mental (e.g. counting up to a certain number).

- Thoughts and acts are not pleasurable but often give a feeling of relief.
- May have 'magical thinking' believing that compulsions are preventing harm to themselves or others.
- Realize that thoughts are their own but unable to stop them.
- Obsessions and compulsions are resisted, often unsuccessfully.

- Autonomic symptoms often felt as tension without physical manifestations.
- Actions may be obvious or covert and hidden.
- May be mild and manageable or severe, interfering with every aspect of the person's life.
- Thoughts may be of a sexual or violent nature but this is common and not always a cause for concern.
- Compulsions may be linked to obsessions for example, 'if I turn the light off and on 50 times I will no longer have these thoughts'.
- Diagnostic criteria (based on ICD-10):
  - obsessions and compulsions must occur on most days for 2 weeks;
  - the sufferer must try to resist at least one thought or act (unsuccessfully);
  - thought of carrying out the act must not be pleasurable;
  - the repetitive nature of the thoughts and acts must be unpleasant;
  - must recognize thoughts as their own.

SCREENING QUESTIONS

- Do you wash or clean a lot?
- Do you have to go back and check things a lot?
- Do your day-to-day activities take a long time to complete?
- Do you like things to be in a special order and does it upset you if someone changes this?
- Do you have thoughts that keep coming into your head that you would like to stop?
- Do these problems interfere with your life?
- The Yale-Brown Obsessive Compulsive Scale (Y-BOCS) is a questionnaire that can be used to monitor a patient during a course of treatment.

> **MICRO-reference**
> Goodman WK, Price LH, Rasmussen SA, Mazure C, Fleischmann RL, Hill CL *et al*. The Yale-Brown Obsessive Compulsive Scale. I. Development, use and reliability. *Arch Gen Psychiatry* 1989; **46:** 1006–11

- Also screen for:
  - self-harm/suicide (see Chapter 15 Psychiatric emergencies, Suicide and Self-harm);
  - depression (see Chapter 7 Affective disorders, Depressive episode).

MANAGEMENT

- Psychological therapy:
  - CBT:

Mental health disorders

- can be individual or group sessions,
- self-help materials can be given;
- exposure and response prevention:
  - a form of CBT involving being exposed to situations that are currently causing anxiety, for example getting hands dirty then lengthening the time before the compulsive ritual is carried out.
- Pharmacological therapy:
  - SSRIs:
    - can be used alone or with CBT,
    - the usual dose to treat OCD is two to three times higher than the usual dose to treat depressive disorder,
    - the minimum mean daily dosage of one of the SSRIs is listed as follows: fluvoxamine 150 mg, fluoxetine 40 mg, sertraline 150 mg and paroxetine 40 mg;
  - other treatments:
    - clomipramine can be used if no response to SSRIs,
    - an antipsychotic (e.g. risperidone) can be used if response not optimal.

PROGNOSIS

- Varies depending on response to treatment:
  - if left untreated may become severe and disabling.
- Poor prognostic factors include:
  - strong conviction about the rationality of the obsession;
  - prominent depression;
  - an underlying medical condition.

8.8 ACUTE STRESS REACTION

AETIOLOGY

- Caused by a severe acute stress (e.g. rape, assault, natural catastrophe, multiple bereavement) or a sudden change in the social position and/or network of a person.

CLINICAL FEATURES

- Symptoms occur within an hour of the event and should usually begin to disappear within hours or days.
- Should not last more than 4 weeks.
- Symptoms are mixed and changing (see Table 8.2).

Table 8.2 Symptoms of acute stress reaction.

PHYSICAL	PSYCHOLOGICAL
Palpitations	Daze
Chest pain	Despair
Feeling sick	Anger
Headache	Withdrawal
Abdominal pain	Overactivity

SCREENING QUESTIONS

- What triggered the symptoms?
- How were you before this happened?
- Screen for risk to self (see Chapter 15 Psychiatric emergencies, Suicide).

MANAGEMENT

- Reassure the patient that this can be a normal reaction and that the symptoms are not a sign of physical disease.
- Counselling if available.
- A short course of diazepam if severe (**not** to be repeated).

PROGNOSIS

- Symptoms should resolve within hours or days.

8.9 POST-TRAUMATIC STRESS DISORDER

EPIDEMIOLOGY

- Up to 30% of people experiencing a traumatic event may develop post-traumatic stress disorder (PTSD).
- Male to female ratio: 1:2.
- Can occur in adults and children.

CLINICAL FEATURES

- A delayed or prolonged response to a traumatic event, for example a disaster, combat, violent incident, experience of torture, terrorism or crime.
- There may be latency to onset of weeks or months (rarely more than 6 months) and the disorder follows a fluctuating course.
- Symptoms:
    - **re-experiencing** – flashbacks, nightmares, intrusive thoughts and mental images;
    - **avoidance** – of people and other reminders of the event;

- **hyperarousal** – increased vigilance, irritability, insomnia, problems concentrating and pronounced startle response;
- **emotional numbing** – detachment, lack of interest in activities and unable to experience new feelings.
- Associated with:
  - depression;
  - drug use;
  - alcohol use;
  - anger.

SCREENING QUESTIONS

- Ask if a traumatic event has occurred in the past and give examples.
- Ask about re-experiencing the event.
- Ask about hyperarousal.
- Ask how the patient feels now when things happen (looking for emotional blunting).
- Ask about the timeline of how the condition has developed.
- Screen for:
  - drug use (see Chapter 5 Substance misuse, Assessment of substance misuse);
  - alcohol use (see Chapter 5 Substance misuse, Assessment of substance misuse);
  - depression (see Chapter 7 Affective disorders, Depressive episode).

MANAGEMENT

- If drug or alcohol abuse are present then treat before treating PTSD (see Chapter 5 Substance misuse, Dependence syndrome).
- Psychological therapy:
  - offer trauma-focused CBT;
  - eye movement desensitization and reprogramming (EMDR):
    - while recalling the traumatic event the patient performs a dual attention movement (e.g. lateral eye movement, bilateral hand tapping),
    - aims to give new insight and decrease sensitivity to memories.
- Pharmacological therapy:
  - antidepressants may be used as a second-line therapy if psychological therapies have not improved the condition;
  - hypnotics can be used to manage short-term sleep difficulties.

PROGNOSIS

- In most cases the disorder will resolve over time especially with interventions as above.
- Some patients may go on to have chronic disorder.

Mental health disorders

8.10 ADJUSTMENT DISORDER

AETIOLOGY

- Triggered by stressful life event (e.g. divorce, moving house).
- More likely to develop disorder if existing coping mechanisms are poor or interrupted.

CLINICAL FEATURES

- Onset usually within 1 month of event and normally resolves by 6 months.
- In some cases can persist for up to 2 years.
- Psychological:
  - feeling unable to cope;
  - worry;
  - anxiety;
  - feeling depressed;
  - unable to plan ahead.
- Physical:
  - inability to carry on with daily routine;
  - regression of behaviour in children (e.g. thumb sucking, bed wetting, not speaking);
  - aggressive outbursts.
- Drug and alcohol use may increase.

SCREENING QUESTIONS

- Ask about symptoms, as described in the section on Adjustment disorder, above.
- Has a stressful event occurred?
- Screen for:
  - depression (see Chapter 7 Affective disorders, Depressive episode);
  - anxiety (see the section on Generalized anxiety disorder, above);
  - alcohol/drug abuse (see Chapter 5 Substance misuse, Assessment of substance misuse);
  - risk to self (see Chapter 15 Psychiatric emergencies, Suicide).

MANAGEMENT

- Usually self-limiting.
- Reassurance from general practitioner (GP).
- If prolonged counselling can be offered.
- Comorbid conditions (e.g. depression) should be treated and the diagnosis reviewed accordingly.

Mental health disorders

8.11 SOMATIZATION DISORDER

DEFINITION

- Disorder characterized by recurrent healthcare-seeking behaviour for multiple somatic complaints of long duration.

EPIDEMIOLOGY

- Lifetime risk: 0.2–2%.
- Age of onset: teenage years; certainly before 30 years.
- Male to female ratio: 1:5.
- Associated with certain personality disorders (PDs):
  - avoidant PD;
  - paranoid PD;
  - obsessive–compulsive PD.

AETIOLOGY

- Genetic factors:
  - 10–20% risk if a first-degree relative is a sufferer.
- Biological factors:
  - cytokine dysregulation has been suggested as a cause for clinical features;
  - decreased metabolism in the frontal lobes and non-dominant hemisphere observed in sufferers.
- Home environment:
  - parental teaching of somatization;
  - excess parental anxiety over childhood illnesses;
  - links to physical and sexual abuse in childhood.

CLINICAL FEATURES

- Multiple, recurrent and frequently changing physical symptoms.
- Long history of contact with primary and specialist medical services.
- Numerous negative investigations including inconclusive operations.
- Persistent refusal to accept negative results.
- Investigations may lead to iatrogenic disease (e.g. abdominal adhesions).
- May be dependent on analgesics or sedatives.
- Symptoms from any system, although gastrointestinal and skin are the commonest.
- Symptoms must have been present for ≥ 2 years.
- Patients will have some impairment from symptoms, especially social or to family function.

DIFFERENTIAL DIAGNOSIS

- Need to rule out other physical or psychiatric disorders before diagnosis of a somatoform disorder can be made.
- Multisystem disorders:
  - acute intermittent porphyria, chronic infection, human immunodeficiency virus, hyperparathyroidism, multiple sclerosis, myasthenia gravis, occult neoplasia, systemic lupus erythematosus, thyroid dysfunction.
- Psychiatric disorders:
  - adjustment disorder, anxiety, dementia, mood disorders, Parkinson's disease, psychotic disorders, substance abuse.

MANAGEMENT

- Limit care to one physician to allow for continuity.
- Regular review of patient.
- Psychotherapy; individual or group.
- Need to be aware that there is a possibility of the patient having a physical disease in the future.

8.12 HYPOCHONDRIACAL DISORDER

EPIDEMIOLOGY

- Prevalence: 1–5% (variable in different population studies).
- Age of onset: 20–30 years.
- Male to female ratio: 1:1.
- Associated with:
  - GAD (>50% comorbidity);
  - health-care professions.

AETIOLOGY

- Learned healthcare-seeking behaviour from parents.
- Linked to childhood sexual abuse.
- Misinterpretation of physical symptoms because of lower threshold for suspecting illness leads to medical-seeking behaviour.
- Subconscious secondary gain from attention gained when ill reinforces behaviour.

CLINICAL FEATURES

- Persistent belief in the presence of one or more physical disorders underlying presenting symptoms (e.g. headaches being interpreted as a brain tumour).
- Symptoms are focused on one or two systems/organs.

- Patient will ask for investigations that identify a specific disease, such as computed tomography (CT) scan.
- Persistent refusal to accept negative investigations.

DIFFERENTIAL DIAGNOSIS

- As for somatization disorder (see the section on Somatization disorder above).

MANAGEMENT

- Regular review of patient by GP.
- Do not offer investigations unless clinically indicated.
- Psychological therapy:
  - group psychotherapy;
  - CBT;
  - behavioural therapy;
  - hypnosis claimed to be effective.

MICRO-print

Dysmorphophobia (aka body dysmorphic disorder):

- variant of hypochondriacal disorder;
- excess preoccupation with imagined or barely noticeable defect in physical appearance such as size of nose;
- leads to significant distress and dysfunction;
- patient may undergo plastic surgery to correct the perceived defect.

8.13 SOMATOFORM AUTONOMIC DYSFUNCTION

CLINICAL FEATURES

- Symptoms of autonomic arousal (e.g. sweating, palpitations or flushing).
- Patient is preoccupied with concern about having a disease within a system under autonomic control (e.g. in cardiovascular system, gastrointestinal system or respiratory system).
- Persistent refusal to accept negative investigations.

8.14 SOMATOFORM PAIN DISORDER

EPIDEMIOLOGY

- High comorbidity with:
  - depression;

- personality disorders;
- substance abuse.
- High prevalence in pain clinics and within surgical specialties.

AETIOLOGY

- Usually associated with stress.

CLINICAL FEATURES

- Persistent, severe and distressing pain.
- Pain cannot be explained by physiological processes or any physical disorder.
- Often there are numerous other symptoms from other systems.

MANAGEMENT

- Analgesics, sedatives and anxiolytics are often ineffective and can lead to dependence.
- Refer to pain clinic as can get some relief from biofeedback or transcutaneous electrical nerve stimulation (TENS).
- Psychological therapy:
  - psychodynamic psychotherapy;
  - hypnosis may be effective.
- Antidepressants may be of use.

MICRO-print

Factitious disorder:

- aka Munchhausen's syndrome;
- intentional feigning or production of symptoms or signs;
- may self-harm or contaminate samples in order to gain medical attention;
- absence of any physical or mental disorder;
- patient wants to play the sick role.

Malingering:

- intentional feigning or production of symptoms or signs in order to gain secondary benefits (e.g. housing, disability living allowance or sick leave);
- comparatively common in legal and military settings.

Munchhausen's syndrome by proxy:

- intentional feigning or production of symptoms or signs in another person (usually a child) under the care of the individual (usually the mother). It is a form of child abuse;
- think of Mischa Barton's character in *The Sixth Sense*.

9 Behavioural syndromes associated with physiological disturbance

9.1 EATING DISORDERS

ANOREXIA NERVOSA

- Definition:
  - deliberate weight loss induced and/or sustained by the patient;
  - fear of fatness with a distorted body image;
  - body mass index (BMI) <17.5;
  - amenorrhoea, or in men, loss of sexual interest and potency.
- Epidemiology:
  - prevalence: 0.1–0.2% of women;
  - male to female ratio: 1:19;
  - peak age of onset 15–19 years;
  - increased incidence in higher socio-economic class.
- Risk factors:
  - female gender;
  - regular excessive exercise;
  - certain occupations:
    - ballet dancers,
    - modelling;
  - comorbid disorders:
    - depression,
    - substance misuse,
    - certain personality disorders, particularly borderline personality disorder.
- Aetiology:
  - a dysfunction of the 5-hydroxytryptamine (5-HT) neurotransmitter system;
  - social opinion that thinness is attractive;
  - personality traits:
    - perfectionism,
    - low self-esteem,
    - obsessive behaviour.

- Clinical features:
  - core features:
    - deliberate weight loss by:
      - diet restriction,
      - excessive exercising,
      - self-induced vomiting,
      - appetite suppressants or diuretics,
      - laxatives;
    - BMI <17.5;
    - morbid fear of fatness;
    - distorted body image;
    - reduced libido;
    - obsessive–compulsive traits.
  - symptoms and signs (see Fig. 9.1).
- Investigations:
  - to rule out differential diagnoses and assess the metabolic consequences of anorexia nervosa; see Table 9.1.
- Differential diagnosis:
  - diabetes mellitus;
  - bulimia nervosa;
  - Addison's disease;
  - malabsorption:
    - coeliac disease,
    - inflammatory bowel disease;
  - malignancy (unlikely).
- Management:
  - correct any medical complications (may require admission);

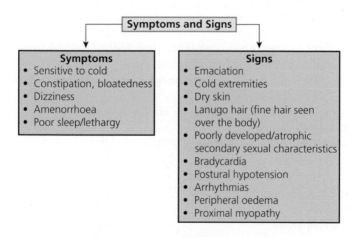

Fig. 9.1 Symptoms and signs of anorexia nervosa.

Mental health disorders

Table 9.1 Investigations in anorexia nervosa.

INVESTIGATION	TEST	COMMON FINDINGS
Bloods	Full blood count	Anaemia: iron deficiency; folate deficiency; B_{12} deficiency
	Urea and electrolytes	Hypokalaemia
	Liver function tests	Hepatitis: raised AST; raised ALT
	Amylase	Raised, owing to pancreatitis
	Lipids	Hypercholesterolaemia
	Glucose	Hypoglycaemia
	Thyroid function tests	Low T_3 with normal TSH and low to normal T_4
	Calcium, magnesium and phosphate	Hypocalcaemia, hypomagnesaemia and hypophosphataemia
	LH, FSH and oestradiol	Low LH, FSH and oestradiol
	Cortisol and growth hormone	Raised cortisol and GH levels
ECG	12-lead ECG	Prolonged QT interval, arrhythmias
Bone density	DEXA scan	Osteopenia, osteoporosis

ALT, alanine aminotransferase; AST, aspartate aminotransferase; DEXA, dual energy X-ray absorptiometry; ECG, electrocardiogram; FSH, follicle-stimulating hormone; GH, growth hormone; LH, luteinizing hormone; T_3, triiodothyronine; T_4, thyroxine; TSH, thyroid-stimulating hormone.

- admit to a psychiatric unit if very low BMI or suicidal (may need detaining under the Mental Health Act):
  - BMI <13.5, risk of death owing to fatal arrhythmia or hypoglycaemia is high;
- refeeding via a nasogastric tube may be necessary.
- Psychological therapy:
  - cognitive behavioural therapy (CBT);
  - interpersonal psychotherapy;
  - focal psychodynamic therapy;
  - family therapy.
- Complications:
  - osteoporosis;
  - hypoglycaemia;

- hypokalaemia leads to:
  - cardiac arrhythmias,
  - renal failure;
- pancreatitis;
- hepatitis;
- seizures;
- peripheral neuropathies;
- refeeding syndrome.
- Prognosis:
  - 20% recover fully;
  - 45% improve partially or fluctuate;
  - 20% suffer chronically;
  - 15% mortality.

BULIMIA NERVOSA

- Definition:
  - uncontrolled binge eating;
  - purging:
    - vomiting,
    - laxatives;
  - preoccupation with body weight and shape;
  - fluctuating body weight:
    - normal,
    - excessive.
- Epidemiology:
  - prevalence: 1–3%;
  - male to female ratio: 1:10;
  - normal age of onset 15–30 years.
- Risk factors:
  - depression;
  - self-harm;
  - substance misuse;
  - personal and family history of obesity;
  - socio-cultural pressure.
- Clinical features:
  - normal or excessive weight which often fluctuates;
  - excessive vomiting;
  - acute oesophageal tears during vomiting;
  - self-loathing;
  - depression;
  - examination findings:
    - weight may be normal,

- signs of vomiting:
  - ○ dental erosions,
  - ○ finger calluses,

MICRO-facts

Russell's sign: calluses on the dorsum of the hand caused by excessive self-induced vomiting.

  - ○ parotid swelling,
  - ○ facial telangiectases;
  - menstrual abnormalities.
- Investigations:
  - as for anorexia nervosa (see the section on Eating disorders above).
- Differential diagnosis:
  - anorexia nervosa.
- Management:
  - nearly all are managed as outpatients;
  - correct any medical abnormalities;
  - psychological therapy:
    - CBT,
    - interpersonal psychotherapy;
  - pharmacological therapy:
    - selective serotonin re-uptake inhibitor (SSRI) antidepressants (see Chapter 13 Pharmacotherapy, Antidepressants) have an antibulimic effect separate from the antidepressant effect:
      - ○ fluoxetine.
- Complications:
  - hypokalaemia can lead to:
    - cardiac arrhythmias,
    - renal failure;
  - oesophageal tears (Mallory–Weiss tears);
  - oesophagitis due to induced vomiting;
  - self-loathing and depression.
- Prognosis:
  - majority make a full recovery;
  - poor prognosis if associated with:
    - depression,
    - high frequency of purging,
    - those with a low BMI,
    - personality disorder,
    - substance misuse,
    - severe or long duration of symptoms.

9.2 SLEEP DISORDERS

THE SLEEP CYCLE

See Table 9.2 for the stages of sleep.

Table 9.2 **The stages of sleep.**

	STAGES OF SLEEP	LENGTH	FEATURES
Non-REM	1. Transition to sleep	5 minutes	Easily wakened
	2. Light sleep	10–25 minutes	True sleep, heart rate slows, eye movements stop
	3. Deep sleep	30–60 minutes	Difficult to awake from, feel groggy and disorientated. Sleep walking occurs in this stage
REM	4. Dream sleep	Variable	Dreams occur. Eyes move rapidly, breathing is shallow and limbs are paralysed

REM, rapid eye movement.

INSOMNIA

- Definition:
    - difficulty in getting to sleep, staying asleep, early waking or non-restorative sleep despite adequate time for rest;
    - leads to daytime tiredness, poor concentration and mood disturbance.
- Aetiology:
    - idiopathic – begins in childhood;
    - stress – environmental, psychosocial, acute (e.g. death of a loved one);
    - psychiatric – mood, anxiety, psychotic disorders, post-traumatic stress disorder (PTSD);
    - medical:
        - cardiovascular (e.g. angina, heart failure),
        - respiratory e.g. chronic obstructive pulmonary disease (COPD), asthma, obstructive sleep apnoea (OSA),
        - dementia,
        - thyroid dysfunction,
        - gastrointestinal (e.g. reflux),
        - genito-urinary (e.g. nocturia, benign prostatic hyperplasia),
        - rheumatology (e.g. fibromyalgia, rheumatoid arthritis),

- chronic pain,
- other (e.g. restless legs syndrome, sleep apnoea);
- drug misuse:
  - alcohol, caffeine, nicotine, illicit drugs,
  - prescribed/over-the-counter medication.
- Clinical features:
  - classification:
    - short term: 1–4 weeks,
    - long term: >4 weeks,
    - primary: no comorbidity,
    - secondary: with a comorbidity or causative factor (see above);
  - difficulty sleeping;
  - daytime symptoms interfering with ability to function;
  - 80% of patients presenting with insomnia have a comorbidity.

MICRO-print

Circadian rhythm disorders are caused by an altered sleep–wake cycle, either intrinsic or caused by shift work or jet lag. Patients have problems going to sleep or getting up at a normal time.

- Screening questions:
  - What is your sleep pattern?
  - What do you believe to be a normal sleep pattern?
  - Is there any impact on daytime life and activities including driving?
  - Assess for comorbidities (see above);
  - How long has this been going on for?
  - Is this a recurring problem?
  - Ask about night-time routine to assess environmental problems (e.g. shift work, noise, young children).
- Investigations:
  - physical causes must be excluded;
  - investigate based on symptoms and history;
  - important to exclude OSA (ask about snoring and other symptoms):
    - record Epworth sleepiness score,
    - refer for sleep studies if appropriate.
- Management:
  - if a comorbidity is present treat as appropriate;
  - if primary insomnia then address sleep hygiene;

> **MICRO-facts**
>
> **Sleep hygiene**
> - Go to bed at the same time every night and get out of bed at the same time every morning.
> - Create a comfortable and relaxing environment (no TV).
> - Use the bed only for sex and sleeping, not working etc.
> - Don't nap during the day.
> - Don't have any caffeine or other stimulants up to 4 hours before going to bed.
> - Avoid large meals and fluids before bed.
> - Do not check the time during the night (i.e. avoid having a bright clock).

- if no improvement with sleep hygiene changes, a 2-week course of a hypnotic drug may be prescribed:
    - benzodiazepines (temazepam, loprazolam, lormetazepam) – short-term use only,
    - non-benzodiazepines (zopiclone, zolpidem, zaleplon),
    - there is no difference between the two types in terms of efficacy,
    - if one hypnotic is not successful another should not be tried.
  - psychological therapies can also be tried (refer for appropriate advice on therapy choice).
- Prognosis:
  - symptoms persist for many years in a substantial number of patients;
  - if the underlying comorbidity is addressed well the condition may improve.

HYPERSOMNIAS OF CENTRAL ORIGIN

- Definition:
  - daytime sleepiness that is not caused by disturbed sleep or misaligned circadian rhythms.
- Narcolepsy:
  - epidemiology:
    - prevalence: 25–50 per 100 000,
    - male to female ratio: 1:1;
  - aetiology:
    - loss of the neuroexcitatory neuropeptide orexin (also known as hypocretin);
  - clinical features:
    - daytime sleepiness,

Mental health disorders

- cataplexy:
  ○ loss of muscle tone,
- hypnagogic hallucinations,
- sleep paralysis:
  ○ complete inability to move for 2 minutes after waking;
- investigations:
  - referral to specialist centre.

PARASOMNIAS

- This group includes:
  - arousal disorders (e.g. sleepwalking and night terrors);
  - sleep–wake transition disorders (e.g. rhythmic movement disorder and sleep talking);
  - parasomnias associated with rapid eye movement (REM) (e.g. nightmares and sleep talking).
- Some of these are discussed below.
- Sleep or night terrors:
  - epidemiology:
    - most common in young children, onset around 3 years of age,
    - usually grow out of the condition by adolescence,
    - may occur in adults;
  - clinical features:
    - arousal during non-REM sleep,
    - there may be shouting, screaming and panic,
    - the patient may be confused and disorientated and have no knowledge of what has happened,
    - the patient will then normally return to sleep,
    - there will be no recall in the morning.
  - management:
    - stay with the child to make sure they do not hurt themselves,
    - do not wake them up,
    - if occurring at the same time each night waking the child beforehand may break the cycle.
- Sleepwalking (somnambulism)
  - epidemiology:
    - occurs mostly in children who will grow out of the disorder,
    - may occur in adults and tends to be a more chronic problem;
  - aetiology:
    - episodes can increase if the person is sleep deprived;
  - clinical features:
    - during non-REM sleep the person will perform complex motor activities, including:
      ○ talking,

○ eating,
○ walking,
○ work-related activity,
○ sexual behaviour;
– the person will appear to be awake;
– there is no recollection of night-time activities the next morning.

9.3 PSYCHOSEXUAL DISORDERS

LACK/LOSS OF DESIRE

- Definition:
  - lack of desire is the main problem and is not secondary to dyspareunia or other problems;
  - does not stop sexual activity but makes initiation less likely.
- Aetiology:
  - organic:
    – any illness,
    – medications,
    – endocrine problems,
    – menopause;
  - psychological:
    – depression,
    – stress;
  - other:
    – relationship problems,
    – life changes (e.g. becoming a mother),
    – lack of sexual knowledge.
- Assessment:
  - take a full history including medical, psychiatric, sexual and relationship;
  - check any medications and side-effects;
  - interview sexual partner (with consent).
- Investigations:
  - necessary to exclude organic causes.
- Management:
  - CBT: to address unhelpful thinking patterns;
  - psychological: to address past experiences;
  - couple: to address relationship issues;
  - behavioural:
    – either as a couple or an individual,
    – focuses on finding sexual likes and desires,
    – become aware of own sexual needs.

Mental health disorders

ORGASMIC DYSFUNCTION

- Definition:
  - persistent or recurrent delay in orgasm or an absence of orgasm.
- Aetiology:
  - lack of desire;
  - inhibitions;
  - poor sexual technique/knowledge;
  - physical illness;
  - side-effects of medication;
  - anxiety/guilt/depression;
  - relationship problems.
- Management:
  - education:
    - sexual technique,
    - normal pathway to orgasm;
  - psychological therapies:
    - couple therapy,
    - sexual therapy;
  - sexual aids:
    - vibrators, lubrication, etc.

PREMATURE EJACULATION

- Aetiology:
  - anxiety;
  - inexperience;
  - hypersensitivity.
- Screening questions:
  - How long does it usually take before ejaculation occurs?
  - Is this always the case?
  - Does it bother you or your partner?
  - How long do you feel would be acceptable before ejaculation?
  - What are your feelings and expectations about the problem?
- Management:
  - psychosexual therapy:
    - couple,
    - individual;
  - relaxation techniques can be useful;
  - pharmacological therapy:
    - SSRIs,
    - topical anaesthetics (can be used inside a condom).

> **MICRO-facts**
>
> Techniques to prevent premature ejaculation:
>
> Stop–start technique. learn when ejaculation is going to occur and control the sexual experience.
> Squeeze technique: squeeze below the head of the penis to prevent ejaculation.

DYSPAREUNIA

- Definition:
  - a recurrent or persistent genital pain associated with sexual intercourse.
- Aetiology:
  - physical factors:
    - infection,
    - circumcision,
    - poor lubrication,
    - atrophic vagina post-menopause;
  - psychological factors:
    - previous painful experience,
    - rape or sexual abuse,
    - poor sexual understanding,
    - insufficient relaxation;
  - factors related to the relationship:
    - poor technique.
- Investigations:
  - exclude physical causes;
  - examination should always be carried out by a specialist.
- Management:
  - education may be sufficient;
  - psychological therapy:
    - couple therapy,
    - sexual therapy.

VAGINISMUS

- Definition:
  - a recurrent or persistent involuntary spasm of the lower third of the vagina that interferes with sexual intercourse.

- Aetiology:
  - fear of pregnancy;
  - fear of intimacy and lack of control;
  - expectation of pain or bleeding;
  - poor sex education (e.g. belief that there is no end to vagina);
  - rape or sexual abuse.
- Management:
  - desensitization with trainers (cones of increasing sizes);
  - individual counselling;
  - education;
  - sexual therapy.

ERECTILE DYSFUNCTION

- Epidemiology:
  - twice as common in men aged over 50 years.
- Aetiology:
  - physical factors:
    - diabetes mellitus,
    - spinal cord injury,
    - renal failure,
    - heart failure;
  - side-effects of medication;
  - psychological factors:
    - anxiety,
    - depression.
- Clinical features:
  - four types:
    - full erection occurs during intercourse but declines before ejaculation,
    - erection does occur but only at times when intercourse is not being considered,
    - partial but not full erection occurs,
    - no erection occurs at all.
- Treatment:
  - psychological therapy:
    - behavioural therapy:
      ○ sensate focus is suitable for patients with performance anxiety,
      ○ it focuses on communication and exploration followed by genital touching and intercourse;
  - pharmacotherapy:
    - phosphodiesterase type 5 inhibitors (PDE5) such as sildenafil (Viagra):
      ○ taken orally before intercourse,

    ○ enhances the effect of nitric oxide,
    ○ side-effects include headache, flushing and impaired vision.

GENDER IDENTITY DISORDERS

> **MICRO-facts**
>
> Gender identity disorders are strictly speaking disorders of adult personality and behaviour, as defined by the ICD-10 and not disorders related to physiological disturbance. They are included here purely for completion in keeping with the theme of this section (i.e. disorders related to sex).

> **MICRO-reference**
>
> http://apps.who.int/classifications/icd10/browse/2010/en

- Trans-sexualism:
  - a desire to live and be accepted as a member of the opposite sex;
  - trans-sexual identity must have been present persistently for at least 2 years;
  - may wish to undergo hormone treatment and surgery to fit with new gender.
- Dual role transvestism:
  - wearing clothes of the other gender for part of the individual's existence but no desire to become a member of the other sex;
  - not linked with sexual excitement (unlike fetishistic transvestitism).

DISORDERS OF SEXUAL PREFERENCE

Table 9.3 features some disorders, although there are many more that are not included.

9.4 DISORDERS RELATED TO THE PUERPERIUM AND MENSTRUATION

POSTPARTUM BLUES

> **MICRO-facts**
>
> It is important to stress to the woman and her family that this is entirely normal.

Table 9.3 Features of disorders of sexual preference.

DISORDER	FEATURES
Fetishism	Reliance on non-living object for sexual arousal (e.g. leather, latex)
Exhibitionism	A recurrent tendency to expose genitalia to strangers in public
Voyeurism	A recurrent tendency to watch people engaging in sexual or intimate behaviour, such as undressing, without their knowledge
Sadomasochism	A preference for sexual activity involving bondage or the infliction of pain and humiliation
Frotteurism	Sexual gratification from rubbing against a non-consenting person

- Also known as baby blues, third-day blues or maternity blues.
- Epidemiology:
  - occurs in up to 50% of mothers.
- Aetiology:
  - fall in oestrogen, progesterone and prolactin roughly 72 hours after birth;
  - not associated with any past medical history of mental disorders.
- Clinical features:
  - can occur at any point within the first 10 days of the puerperium;
  - peaks at days 3–5;
  - weepiness not necessarily related to any specific cause;
  - emotional lability;
  - irritability;
  - sleep disturbance;
  - anxiety.
- Management:
  - the disorder is self-limiting so reassurance is all that is needed.
- Prognosis:
  - usually lasts days to weeks;
  - if severely affected it can lead to postnatal depression (see section on Postnatal depression below).

POSTNATAL DEPRESSION

- Epidemiology:
  - incidence: 10–15% of mothers.

- Risk factors:
  - personal or family history of depression;
  - past history of bipolar affective disorder;
  - recent stressful life events;
  - young maternal age;
  - single or marital difficulties;
  - lack of close confiding relationship;
  - poor relationship with own mother;
  - unwanted pregnancy.
- Clinical features:
  - occurs within 6 months of delivery;
  - similar features to depressive episode (see Chapter 7 Affective disorders, Depressive episode);
  - actual suicide is rare;
  - anxious preoccupation with infant's health;
  - decreased affection for infant;
  - infanticidal thoughts.

MICRO-facts

It is important to establish whether infanticidal thoughts are **ego-dystonic** (repulsive to mother) or **ego-syntonic** (entertained by mother).

- Management:
  - use of the Edinburgh Postnatal Depression Scale (EPDS) to identify mothers at risk;
  - screening should be done by general practitioner (GP) and health visitor on postnatal baby checks;

MICRO-print
Edinburgh Postnatal Depression Scale
Consists of 10 statements concerning the previous 7 days. Respondents select one of the following four options for each statement depending on how they have been feeling:
1. Yes, all the time.
2. Yes, most of the time.
3. No, not very often.
4. No, not at all.
Statements:
1. I have been able to laugh and see the funny side of things.
2. I have looked forward with enjoyment to things.
3. I have blamed myself unnecessarily when things go wrong.

continued...

Mental health disorders

continued...

4. I have been anxious or worried for no good reason.
5. I have felt scared or panicky for no very good reason.
6. Things have been getting on top of me.
7. I have been so unhappy that I have had difficulty sleeping.
8. I have felt sad or miserable.
9. I have been so unhappy that I have been crying.
10. The thought of harming myself has occurred to me.

For statements 1, 2 and 4: option 1 scores 0, option 2 scores 1, option 3 scores 2 and option 4 scores 3. For the rest of the statements: option 1 scores 3, option 2 scores 2, option 3 scores 1 and option 4 scores 0. A total score of ≥10 indicates possible depression (original source Cox *et al.* 1987)

MICRO-reference

Cox JL, Holden JM, and Sagovsky R. Detection of postnatal depression: development of the 10-item Edinburgh Postnatal Depression Scale. *Br J Psychiatry* 1987; **150**: 782–6.

- may need hospitalization if risk of self-harm or infanticide;
- psychological therapy:
  - individual counselling,
  - couples therapy;
- pharmacological therapy:
  - consider antidepressants if severe (seek specialist advice because some antidepressants are contraindicated for breastfeeding),
  - tricyclic antidepressants are widely used and are relatively safe,
  - selective serotonin reuptake inhibitors may be safer if the patient is at high risk of overdose,
  - need to caution if breastfeeding,
  - typically prescribed for 6 months, although can continue for up to 1 year if severe,
  - can give an antidepressant as prophylaxis in future pregnancies.

PUERPERAL PSYCHOSIS

- Epidemiology:
  - incidence rate: 0.1–0.2%.
- Risk factors:
  - primiparity;

- instrumental birth;
- personal or family history of a psychiatric disorder;
- lack of social support.

MICRO-facts

Puerperal psychosis is more closely related to bipolar affective disorders (especially depressive presentations) than any of the psychotic disorders.

- Clinical features:
  - occurs 1–2 weeks after delivery;
  - early symptoms:
    - fatigue,
    - insomnia,
    - restlessness,
    - emotional lability,
    - perplexity;
  - later symptoms:
    - suspiciousness,
    - confusion,
    - incoherence,
    - irrationality,
    - delusions of infant's death,
    - delusions of persecution,
    - obsessive concern about infant's health,
    - command hallucinations,
    - infanticidal thoughts,
    - suicidal thoughts,
    - patients often have one or more of Schneider's first-rank symptoms of schizophrenia (see Chapter 6 Schizophrenia and delusional disorders, Schizophrenia).
- Management:
  - urgent risk assessment of mother to baby needs to be carried out;
  - urgent admission to hospital if available to mother and baby unit;
  - detention under the Mental Health Act may be necessary;
  - pharmacological therapy:
    - antipsychotics or antidepressants as for normal treatment of similar episodes (see Chapter 6 Schizophrenia and delusional disorders, Schizophrenia and Chapter 7 Affective disorders, Depressive episode);
  - good evidence for efficacy of electroconvulsive therapy (ECT).

Mental health disorders

- Prognosis:
  - up to two-thirds of sufferers will have a second affective episode within baby's first year;
  - one in three chance of recurrence after subsequent childbirth;
  - better prognosis if supportive family environment.

MICRO-print
Prescribing during pregnancy

Antidepressants:

- Most clinical experience is with tricyclic antidepressants (TCAs) (rather than SSRIs).
- Safest SSRI to prescribe is fluoxetine.
- Paroxetine is associated with fetal cardiac defects.
- Neonatal discontinuation syndrome after use of paroxetine (convulsions, agitation and irritability).
- SSRI use late in pregnancy is associated with persistent pulmonary hypertension of the newborn (PPHN).

Mood stabilizers:

- An antipsychotic would be preferable to an anticonvulsant for mood stabilization in pregnancy.
- Lithium is associated with congenital heart defects and Ebstein's anomaly; therefore, **do not** prescribe during pregnancy or breastfeeding.
- Valproate and carbamazepine are associated with neural tube defects in neonate.
- Lamotrigine is associated with cleft palate.

Benzodiazepines:

- Associated with cleft palate and floppy baby syndrome in the neonate.

Antipsychotics:

- Most clinical experience is with typicals (chlorpromazine, haloperidol and trifluoperazine).
- Raised prolactin levels may affect fertility.
- Risk of extrapyramidal symptoms in the breastfed infant.

MICRO-reference
National Institute for Health and Clinical Excellence. *Antenatal and postnatal mental health. CG45.* London: National Institute for Health and Clinical Excellence, 2007.

PREMENSTRUAL SYNDROME

- Epidemiology:
  - 40% of women experience symptoms of premenstrual syndrome (PMS);
  - 5% meet the criteria of PMS with impairment in functioning;
  - 30–40% of women with PMS have depressive disorder.
- Clinical features:
  - marked depression;
  - anxiety;
  - anger;
  - affective lability;
  - reduction in interest;
  - difficulty in concentrating;
  - lethargy and lack of energy;
  - overeating;
  - hypersomnia or insomnia;
  - feeling overwhelmed;
  - breast tenderness;
  - headache;
  - muscle pain.
- Management:
  - psychological therapy:
    - CBT;
  - pharmacological therapy:
    - SSRIs (e.g. sertraline);
  - lifestyle changes:
    - carbohydrate-rich diet,
    - increased dietary fibre,
    - exercise,
    - relaxation techniques.

Disorders of adult personality

10.1 DEFINITION

- DSM-IV defines personality disorder (PD) as enduring subjective experiences and behaviour that:
    - deviate from cultural standards;
    - are rigidly pervasive;
    - have an onset in adolescence or early adulthood;
    - are stable through time;
    - lead to unhappiness and impairment;
    - is not caused by another mental disorder or substance abuse (although either of these may be present concurrently).

> **MICRO-reference**
> American Psychiatric Association. *Diagnostic and statistical manual of mental disorders*, 4th edn (text revision). Washington, DC: American Psychiatric Association, 2000.

10.2 EPIDEMIOLOGY

- Prevalence in general population: 4–13%.
- Prevalence in patients with a concurrent psychiatric disorder: $\sim 50\%$.
- Male to female ratio: male > female.

10.3 AETIOLOGY

- Mostly unknown.

GENETIC FACTORS

- Higher concordance rates in monozygotic twins over dizygotic twins, irrespective of whether they were raised in the same environment.
- Cluster A personality disorders are more common in first-degree relatives of patients with schizophrenia.

BIOLOGICAL FACTORS

- High levels of testosterone, oestrone and 17-oestradiol in patients with impulsive behaviour.
- Low levels of the serotonin metabolite 5-hydroxyindoleacetic acid (5-HIAA) have been reported in patients with suicidal or aggressive behaviour.
- Selective serotonin re-uptake inhibitors (SSRIs) have been shown to modify negative personality traits associated with depression (e.g. neuroticism and extraversion).

PSYCHOANALYTICAL THEORY

- Freud describes personality disorders as failure to progress through the stages of psychosexual development.
- This leads to the use of defence mechanisms that manifest as personality disorders.

10.4 CLASSIFICATION

CLUSTER A – THE PARANOID TYPE

- Also known as odd or eccentric.
- Consists of paranoid, schizoid and schizotypal PD (Table 10.1).

CLUSTER B – THE DRAMATIC TYPE

- Also known as dramatic, emotional or erratic.
- Consists of antisocial, borderline, histrionic and narcissistic PD (Table 10.2).

CLUSTER C – THE ANXIOUS TYPE

- Also known as anxious or fearful.
- Consists of avoidant, dependent and obsessive–compulsive (anankastic) PD (Table 10.3).

> **MICRO-print**
> The three clusters (A, B and C) used to be referred to as MAD, BAD and SAD clusters, respectively. This is not only inappropriate but also reinforces negative stereotypes and further stigmatizes individuals with mental health difficulties.

Mental health disorders

Table 10.1 Features of cluster A personality disorders.

PERSONALITY DISORDER	SPECIFIC EPIDEMIOLOGY	SPECIFIC AETIOLOGY	CLINICAL FEATURES
Paranoid	0.5–2.5% prevalence Male > female More common in lower socioeconomic classes	More common in first-degree relatives of schizophrenics Defence mechanism: projection of negative internal feelings onto others	Suspicious Mistrustful Resentful Bears grudges Jealous (especially sexual) Self-important Sensitive
Schizoid	0.5–1.5% prevalence Male:female = 2:1 More common in offender populations	More common in first-degree relatives of schizophrenics Defence mechanism: excessive use of fantasy	Emotionally cold No desire for relationships (platonic or sexual) Does not enjoy activities Unsociable Excess introspection and fantasy
Schizotypal	3% prevalence Male > female	More common in first-degree relatives of schizophrenics Linked to dopamine dysregulation	'Magical thinking' (e.g. belief in clairvoyance) Odd behaviour Eccentric appearance Ideas of reference Paranoid ideations Suspicious Socially withdrawn Vague or circumstantial thinking

Table 10.2 Features of cluster B personality disorders.

PERSONALITY DISORDER	SPECIFIC EPIDEMIOLOGY	SPECIFIC AETIOLOGY	CLINICAL FEATURES
Antisocial	3% male prevalence 1% female prevalence 75% prevalence in prisons Onset usually before 15 years High comorbidity with substance abuse and conduct disorder More common in urban settings	EEG shows slow wave activity Reduced grey matter volume in the prefrontal cortex, which has been suggested as a cause for the low arousal, poor fear conditioning, lack of conscience and decision-making deficits shown by these patients	Callous lack of concern for others Lack of remorse Lack of guilt Transient relationships Repeated unlawful or aggressive behaviour Impulsive Repeated lying Reckless irresponsibility Irritability
Borderline	1–2% prevalence Male:female = 1:2 Young age of onset 9% suicide rate High comorbidity with depression, PTSD, substance abuse and bulimia nervosa	High rate of early abuse (sexual, physical and emotional) More common in first-degree relatives of patients with depression EEG shows slow wave activity Defence mechanisms: (1) splitting (i.e. adopting a polarized view of the world where people are either all good or all bad); (2) projective identification (i.e. subconscious projecting of self onto others)	Fear of abandonment Unstable intense relationships Unstable self-image Unstable fluctuating mood Dangerous impulsivity (e.g. substance abuse, sexual promiscuity or eating disorders) Recurrent self-harm Suicidal ideation Transient stress-related paranoia Aggressive behaviour Transient psychotic episodes ('micropsychosis') Splitting

(Continued)

Mental health disorders

Mental health disorders

Table 10.2 (Continued)

PERSONALITY DISORDER	SPECIFIC EPIDEMIOLOGY	SPECIFIC AETIOLOGY	CLINICAL FEATURES
Histrionic	2–3% prevalence Male < female Comorbidity with somatization disorder and alcohol abuse	Associated with authoritarian or seductive paternal attitudes during childhood Defence mechanism: dissociation or denial	Attention seeking Inappropriate seductive behaviour Shallow labile affect Dramatic Vain Self-absorbed Easily suggestible Views relationships as more intimate than they are
Narcissistic (does not exist in the ICD-10)	Less than 1% prevalence Male > female More common in offender settings	Narcissism has been suggested to be a defence against the awareness of low self-esteem	Grandiose self-importance Need for admiration Exploitation of others Lack of empathy Arrogant Haughty Envious but believes others envy them

EEG, electroencephalogram; PTSD, post-traumatic stress disorder.

Table 10.3 Features of cluster C personality disorders.

PERSONALITY DISORDER	SPECIFIC EPIDEMIOLOGY	SPECIFIC AETIOLOGY	CLINICAL FEATURES
Avoidant	1–10% prevalence Male:female = 1:1 Comorbidity with social phobia	Avoidant behaviour has been suggested to be an expression of extreme introversion and neuroticism	Tense Feeling of social inferiority Subsequent social inhibition Preoccupation with rejection Hypersensitivity to critical remarks Avoids involvement in relationships
Dependent	1–2.5% prevalence Comorbidity with borderline personality disorder	Insecure attachment Parents who prohibit independence	Submissive Clinging Needs others to make decisions for them Fear that unable to care for self Fears separation as feels helpless when not in a relationship
Obsessive–compulsive (anankastic)	1–2% prevalence Male > female More common in eldest children, Caucasians and in high socioeconomic classes	More common in first-degree relatives of sufferers of obsessive–compulsive personality disorder Defence mechanism: isolation	Preoccupation with rules, details, lists and organization Perfectionism Rigid thinking Stubborn Indecisive Excess dedication to work Unable to delegate Overly cautious

Mental health disorders

> **MICRO-references**
>
> National Institute for Health and Clinical Excellence. *Antisocial personality disorder. CG77.* London: National Institute for Health and Clinical Excellence, 2009.
>
> National Institute for Health and Clinical Excellence. *Borderline personality disorder. CG78.* London: National Institute for Health and Clinical Excellence, 2009.

10.5 TREATMENT

- Admission and/or detention under the Mental Health Act may be necessary if presenting a significant risk of harm to self or others.
- Psychological therapy:
    - cluster A:
        - individual cognitive behavioural therapy (CBT) is much more effective than group CBT;
    - cluster B:
        - group CBT is much more effective than individual CBT,
        - cognitive analytical therapy (CAT) is effective in borderline PD,
        - mentalization-based therapy can be effective in borderline PD,
        - dialectical behavioural therapy (DBT) is useful in the case of parasuicidal actions (usually requires 1 year of commitment),
        - behavioural therapy to control impulses, anger and reduce sensitivity to criticism,
        - social skills therapy in borderline PD to identify the effect of actions on others,
        - in borderline PD twice weekly sessions are used for at least 3 months,
        - avoid individual CBT in histrionic PD;
    - cluster C:
        - group CBT is more effective than individual CBT,
        - assertiveness training to build self-confidence and improve social functioning,
        - family therapy in dependent PD,
        - behavioural therapy in obsessive–compulsive PD to develop alternative coping strategies.

> **MICRO-facts**
>
> Cognitive analytical therapy (CAT):
> - Identification of faulty procedures such as traps (repetitive cycles of behaviour and their consequences become perpetuated), dilemma
>
> *continued...*

continued...

(false choices or unduly narrowed options) and snag (extreme pessimism about the future that halts a plan before it even runs).

Mentalization-based therapy:

- Helps patients develop the capacity to recognize the mental states in others as a result of failure in parental responsiveness during their childhood.
- Helps patients to express emotions appropriately and to form a coherent sense of self.

Dialectical behavioural therapy (DBT) – four modes of treatment:

1. Weekly individual psychotherapy.
2. Group skills training with skills acquisition focusing on mindfulness, interpersonal effectiveness, emotional regulation and distress tolerance.
3. Skill coaching phone calls.
4. Therapist consult team meetings.

- Pharmacological therapy:
  - in general only used for comorbid conditions.
  - cluster A:
    - benzodiazepines for agitation or anxiety,
    - antipsychotics for ideas of reference or paranoia,
    - manage comorbid mental health disorders as appropriate;
  - cluster B:
    - do not routinely use medications,
    - if severe anger or impulsivity is interfering with function then consider use of an antipsychotic or antidepressant,
    - if sedative is necessary in borderline PD use an antihistamine to avoid risk of dependence,
    - lithium if mood swings;
  - cluster C:
    - benzodiazepines for intractable anxiety,
    - antidepressants can be useful especially in obsessive–compulsive PD.

10.6 PROGNOSIS

- Generally poor because personality disorders are stable and enduring traits.
- 50% of patients with borderline PD show clinical recovery in 10–25 years.
- Schizotypal PD predisposes to development of schizophrenia.
- Treatment of dependent PD is often very successful, especially if the pathological relationship (dependent partner) is broken.

Mental health disorders

11 Learning disability and child and adolescent disorders

11.1 GENERAL LEARNING DISABILITY

EPIDEMIOLOGY

- Prevalence: ~4%.
- Around 1.5 million people in the UK affected.

AETIOLOGY

Causes of learning disabilities are shown in Fig. 11.1

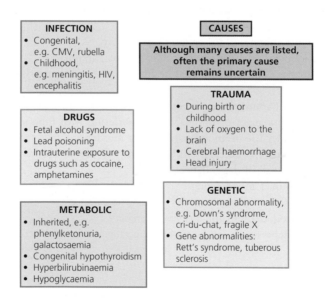

INFECTION
- Congenital, e.g. CMV, rubella
- Childhood, e.g. meningitis, HIV, encephalitis

CAUSES
Although many causes are listed, often the primary cause remains uncertain

DRUGS
- Fetal alcohol syndrome
- Lead poisoning
- Intrauterine exposure to drugs such as cocaine, amphetamines

TRAUMA
- During birth or childhood
- Lack of oxygen to the brain
- Cerebral haemorrhage
- Head injury

METABOLIC
- Inherited, e.g. phenylketonuria, galactosaemia
- Congenital hypothyroidism
- Hyperbilirubinaemia
- Hypoglycaemia

GENETIC
- Chromosomal abnormality, e.g. Down's syndrome, cri-du-chat, fragile X
- Gene abnormalities: Rett's syndrome, tuberous sclerosis

Fig. 11.1 Causes of learning disabilities. CMV, cytomegalovirus; HIV, human immunodeficiency virus.

CLINICAL FEATURES

> **MICRO-facts**
>
> Three main criteria:
> - Onset during childhood.
> - Impairment of social functioning.
> - Impairment of intelligence.

- Depend on the level of impairment.
- Two main features:
  - behavioural phenotypes, these can be syndrome specific (e.g. compulsive self-injuring in Lesch–Nyhan syndrome).
  - challenging behaviours (e.g. violent or inappropriate behaviour).
- Other features:
  - infants may be late in reaching developmental milestones;
  - parental or school concern with achievements and progress;
  - patients may take longer to learn a new task or to adapt to a new environment;
  - may need help with activities of daily living (ADLs).
- Classification of levels of learning disability: see Table 11.1
- Often associated with:
  - physical disorders (e.g. epilepsy, visual impairment).
  - other psychiatric disorders (e.g. autism).

SCREENING QUESTIONS

- Assessment should be undertaken by a multidisciplinary team (MDT) involving patient, family, carers, general practitioner (GP), social worker, paediatrician (if under 18) and a psychiatrist.
- Pregnancy:
  - Any problems/maternal illnesses?
  - Any medications/drugs taken during pregnancy?
- Birth:
  - Was the child born at term?
  - Any problems at birth?
  - Did the baby need special care?
- Childhood:
  - Did the child meet their developmental milestones on time?
  - What was the highest level of development?
  - When were problems first noticed?
  - Were there any childhood illnesses/trauma?

Mental health disorders

Table 11.1 Classification of learning disabilities.

	IQ	COMMUNICATION	MENTAL AGE (YEARS)	EMPLOYMENT	ADLs
Mild	50–69	Normal speech	9–12	Able to work	No help needed
Moderate	35–49	Should develop basic speech	6–9	May work in sheltered employment	May need assistance
Severe	20–34	Little/no speech but may be able to communicate needs	3–6	Unable to work	May have limited ability but will need assistance
Profound	Under 20	Little/no language or understanding	<3	Unable to work	Needs 24-hour support

ADLs, activities of daily living.

- Family history:
  - Does anyone in the family suffer from similar problems?
- Current situation:
  - Any behavioural problems?
  - Any physical problems?
  - How is the patient's sleep and appetite?
  - What is their current living and work situation?
  - Do they require care and if so to what level?
- Psychiatric:
  - screening for depression (see Chapter 7 Affective disorders, Depressive episode), may be difficult and can be expressed through changes in behaviour;
  - screening for anxiety (see Chapter 8 Anxiety and neuroses, Generalized anxiety disorder), may be difficult and can be expressed through changes in behaviour;
  - screen for schizophrenia (see Chapter 6 Schizophrenia and delusional disorders, Schizophrenia), which can be three times more common in patients with lower IQ;
  - assessment for psychiatric comorbidities in individuals with more severe learning disabilities may be very difficult.

MANAGEMENT

- Need appropriate housing (may need sheltered accommodation) with appropriate level of care.
- Need support to find suitable employment.
- If patient is a child, they will need educational support, which may include Statement of Special Educational Needs.
- May need help to access benefits and manage financial affairs.
- If cared for by family it is important to arrange respite care if wanted.
- Prescribing:
  - start with low dose – threshold for experiencing side-effects may be lower;
  - use elderly doses if listed in the *British National Formulary* (BNF);
  - important to monitor patient closely as they may not be able to report side-effects;
  - avoid poly-pharmacy.

> **MICRO-reference**
> Joint Formulary Committee. *British National Formulary*, 61st edn. London: British Medical Association and Royal Pharmaceutical Society, 2011.

PROGNOSIS

- Varies greatly, some patients will require 24-hour care for life and some will live totally independently.

SAFEGUARDING

- Patients with learning difficulties are vulnerable to financial, physical and sexual exploitation.
- Owing to impaired communication they may be unable to make others aware of what is happening to them.
- A change in behaviour with increased aggression, distress or sexualized behaviour may indicate abuse.
- Social workers are often required in the management of learning-disabled individuals to ensure their safeguarding.

11.2 DOWN'S SYNDROME

EPIDEMIOLOGY

- Prevalence: 1 in 800 live births (1 in 80 if mother over 40 years old).

AETIOLOGY

- 94% results from non-dysjunction or trisomy 21.
- 5% results from translocation of chromosome 21.
- 1% results from mosaicism.

CLINICAL FEATURES

- Small round head.
- Brushfield spots on iris.
- Hearing impairment.
- Congenital heart disease.
- Curved little fingers.
- Single palmar crease.
- Learning disability.
- Sandal gap between first and second toes.

PROGNOSIS

- At risk of Alzheimer's disease.
- Hypothyroidism is common.
- Most common cause of death is respiratory infection.

11.3 FRAGILE X SYNDROME

EPIDEMIOLOGY

- Prevalence: 0.01–0.05%.
- Male to female ratio: 1:2–3.
- Most common inherited cause of learning disability.
- 1 in 700 females is a carrier.

AETIOLOGY

- X-linked dominant with low penetrance.

CLINICAL FEATURES

- Macrocephaly.
- Large, floppy ears.
- High, arched palate.
- Prominent jaw.
- Macro-orchidism.
- Cardiac abnormalities.
- Learning disability:
    - mild in females;
    - moderate to severe in males.

11.4 FETAL ALCOHOL SYNDROME

EPIDEMIOLOGY

- Leading non-genetic cause of learning disability in Western countries.

AETIOLOGY

- Alcohol consumption during pregnancy.

CLINICAL FEATURES

- Microcephaly.
- Epicanthal folds.
- Low nasal bridge.
- Mild to moderate learning disability.
- Withdrawal symptoms at birth.
- Growth retardation.

Mental health disorders

11.5 PSYCHIATRIC ASSESSMENT IN CHILDREN

Assessment in child and adolescent psychiatry involves many different members of the young person's family and other members of the multidisciplinary team, such as teachers, educational psychologists, family therapists.

INTERVIEWING THE FAMILY

- Make sure the interviewing room is large enough to accommodate everyone and that all people in the room can be seen by everyone (e.g. sitting in a circle).
- Make sure the room is friendly to young people (e.g. toys, pens and paper).
- Allow each person the chance to introduce themselves to everyone else in the room as young people may attend with other adults, not always mum and dad.
- Try and generate a family tree.
- Allow the family to talk with one another and observe behaviours and attitudes within the family.

INTERVIEWING THE YOUNG PERSON ALONE

- This will depend on the age of the young person and their ability to engage with the interviewer on a one-to-one basis.
- Ask open questions as this gives the chance for the young person to talk more freely.
- Ask them what they think the problem is and what they want to achieve from attending the sessions.
- Start by asking more general questions (e.g. about hobbies and interests) and then try and focus on the problem.

INPUT FROM OTHER PROFESSIONALS

- It may be useful to gain reports about the young person's behaviour from school or nursery.
- Psychological assessment may be necessary.
- Information from the GP or from paediatricians who have seen the young person would also be of value.

11.6 CONDUCT DISORDERS

DEFINITION

Conduct disorder (CD) is a disorder of young people characterized by persistent antisocial, aggressive or defiant behaviours.

EPIDEMIOLOGY

- Prevalence: 4%.
- Male to female ratio: 3:1.

AETIOLOGY/RISK FACTORS

- Parent factors:
  - severe/violent parenting;
  - no boundaries set;
  - divorce;
  - rejection;
  - substance misuse;
  - family feuds.
- Child factors:
  - low IQ;
  - difficult temperament.
  - anxiety/depression.
- Social factors:
  - children who are in the care system;
  - low socioeconomic class.

CLINICAL FEATURES

- Two types:
  - socialized (peer acceptance);
  - unsocialized (peer rejection).
- Features can be reported by the teachers or family and include:
  - disobedience;
  - excessive fighting and bullying;
  - lying;
  - truancy;
  - cruelty to animals or other people;
  - stealing;
  - starting fires and damaging property;
  - inappropriate sexual behaviour.

MICRO-reference
http://apps.who.int/classifications/icd10/browse/2010/en#/F90-F98

- At least three features must be present for 6–12 months to make the diagnosis.

Mental health disorders

INVESTIGATIONS

- Developmental assessment.
- Assessment for educational difficulties (e.g. dyslexia).

MANAGEMENT

- Psychotherapies:
  - art therapy;
  - family therapy;
  - behavioural therapy;
  - group therapy.
- Remedial teaching to address educational needs.
- Parenting management training: to emphasise consistent parenting.
- Alternative peer group activities for the young person.

PROGNOSIS

- Around 30% can develop antisocial personality disorder.
- Poor prognosis associated with:
  - lower socioeconomic group;
  - low IQ;
  - early onset;
  - pervasiveness and associated hyperactivity.

11.7 OPPOSITIONAL DEFIANT DISORDER

- Age of onset: 3–8 years.
- Average duration of symptoms is 6 months.
- Defiant behaviours occur at home and in front of familiar people.
- Features:
  - temper tantrums;
  - anger;
  - argument with adults;
  - defying rules and blaming others.
- Less destructive and less deceitful compared to children with CD.
- Prognosis for children with oppositional defiant disorder (ODD) is better than for those with CD.

11.8 DISORDERS OF SOCIAL FUNCTIONING

- Within this group are the disorders of attachment.
- These disorders develop throughout the developmental period:
  - attachment disorders are present before the age of 5 years.
- The main attachment disorder of childhood is reactive attachment disorder which can then be subdivided into inhibited and disinhibited.

- Features of reactive attachment disorder are:
  - fearfulness;
  - poor social interaction;
  - aggression towards themselves and to others;
  - misery;
  - hypervigilance.

MICRO-print

Normal attachment behaviour (age 6 months to 3 years):

- when attachment figure leaves the room the child will cry, try to follow them and call for them;
- hugging and climbing onto the lap of attachment figure;
- immediately seek contact with attachment figure after separation;
- cling to attachment figure when anxious or afraid.

11.9 HYPERKINETIC DISORDER

DEFINITION

- Hyperkinetic disorder is commonly known as attention-deficit hyperactivity disorder (ADHD).
- Patients demonstrate inattention, impulsivity and over-activity which is present before 6 years of age.

EPIDEMIOLOGY

- Prevalence 2–5%.
- Male to female ratio: 3:1.

AETIOLOGY/RISK FACTORS

- 50% risk in monozygotic twins.
- Increased substance misuse and conduct disorder in the parents.
- Dopamine and noradrenaline dysregulation in the frontal cortex.
- Common comorbidities include:
  - conduct disorder;
  - learning difficulties;
  - antisocial behaviour;
  - depression.

CLINICAL FEATURES

The ICD-10 key diagnostic criteria include:
- Hyperactive and impulsive features:
  - reckless and impulsive;
  - fidgeting;

- breaks the rules;
- interrupts others;
- jumps the queue;
- talks excessively.
- Inattention features:
  - distractibility;
  - inability to listen;
  - forgetful.

INVESTIGATIONS

- Psychometric testing.
- Discuss with parents and teachers to see that features are present in both environments.
- Connor's assessment by teachers and parents.

MANAGEMENT

- Information and support for the parents and teachers.
- Identify educational needs and manage environmental factors.
- Behavioural therapy.
- Psychostimulants such as methylphenidate or dexamphetamine (common side-effects include weight loss, appetite suppression, abdominal pain, headache and tics).
- Non-stimulant: atomoxetine (selective noradrenaline reuptake inhibitor) for young people who develop tics after taking psychostimulants.

PROGNOSIS

- Most features will have reduced by puberty.
- Severe cases may persist into adulthood.
- If comorbidities exist, a poorer prognosis is likely and features may persist.

11.10 AUTISM

DEFINITION

- Pervasive development disorder characterized by impairments in language development, social interaction (e.g. eye contact) and communication.
- Age of onset is before 3 years.

EPIDEMIOLOGY

- Prevalence: 1/770.
- Male to female ratio: 4:1.

Mental health disorders

AETIOLOGY/RISK FACTORS

- Heritability is over 90% with higher concordance in monozygotic twins.
- Lesions in amygdala, corpus callosum and cerebellum.
- Conditions associated with autism include rubella, fragile X syndrome, tuberous sclerosis and phenylketonuria.
- Theory of mind suggests that people with autism lack the capacity to attribute independent mental states to self and others in order to predict and explain actions of other people.

CLINICAL FEATURES

- Abnormal receptive or expressive language.
- Abnormal selective or reciprocal social interaction.
- Abnormal functional or symbolic play.
- Abnormal reciprocal social interactions (e.g. failure in eye gaze and body language).
- Failure in development of peer relationship.
- Lack of socio-emotional reciprocity.
- Lack of spontaneous sharing with other people.
- Lack of development of spoken language.
- Lack of social imitative play.
- Failure to initiate or sustain conversational interchange.
- Stereotyped and repetitive use of language.
- Restricted, stereotyped and repetitive behaviour (e.g. preoccupation with stereotyped interest, compulsive adherence to rituals, motor mannerisms, preoccupation with non-functional elements of toys).

INVESTIGATIONS

- Functional analysis of a child's behaviour.
- Autism Diagnostic Observation Schedule (ADOS) for patient.
- Autism Diagnostic Interview for parents.
- IQ test: performance IQ is better than verbal IQ.

MANAGEMENT

- Special education starting at age 2–3 years.
- Speech and occupational therapy.
- Social skills training.
- Home- and school-based behavioural programmes.
- Parent support.
- Selective serotonin re-uptake inhibitors (SSRIs) for repetitive behaviour.
- Risperidone for aggressive behaviour.

Mental health disorders

PROGNOSIS

- 50% do not develop useful speech.
- 30% develop a seizure disorder.
- 10% are able to work.

11.11 ASPERGER'S SYNDROME

DEFINITION

- A form of pervasive development disorder but unlike autism, language development is normal.

EPIDEMIOLOGY

- Prevalence: 3–4 per 1000 children.
- Male to female ratio: 9:1.

AETIOLOGY/RISK FACTORS

- Right hemisphere lesions.

CLINICAL FEATURES

- Motor clumsiness.
- Fluent speech.
- Preoccupation with restricted, stereotyped and repetitive interests and associated activities.
- Extensive information is often acquired in a mechanical fashion.
- Good with logic, rules and routine.
- Problems distinguishing people of different social roles, as well as recognizing social boundaries (e.g. the patient would talk to the principal and their classmates in the same manner).
- Troubles with normal social conventions.
- Troubles with making and keeping friendships.
- Introverted with less need for friendships.

INVESTIGATIONS

- IQ test: verbal IQs > performance IQs.

MANAGEMENT

- Psychoeducation for parents.
- Maintain routines at home and school.
- Supportive counselling for adolescents.
- Employment in job that emphasizes on routines (e.g. librarian, assembly line workers).

PROGNOSIS

- A strong tendency for the abnormalities to persist into adolescence and adult life.
- Psychotic episodes occasionally occur in early adult life.

11.12 TOURETTE'S SYNDROME

DEFINITION

- Tourette's syndrome is characterized with tics:
  - tics are sudden, rapid and involuntary movements of circumscribed muscles without any purpose.

EPIDEMIOLOGY

- Tourette's syndrome is rare (0.05%).
- Male to female ratio: 3:1.
- 10–25% of children manifest simple tics.

AETIOLOGY/RISK FACTORS

- Association with obsessive compulsive disorder.
- Dopamine excess.
- Provoked by stimulants.

CLINICAL FEATURES

- Onset is before age 18 years.
- Tics occur many times per day, most days for over 12 months without remission for more than 2 months.
- Multiple motor tics.
- Vocal tics include grunting, snarling, coprolalia (swearing) and echolalia (repeating vocalizations of others).
- Absence of neurological disorder.
- Fluctuating course.

TREATMENT

- Antipsychotics treatment (e.g. haloperidol).
- Risperidone and sulpiride are also effective and better tolerated than haloperidol.
- Behaviour therapy (e.g. habit reversal) involves performing simultaneous incompatible movements to reduce unwanted movements.
- Remedial academic assistance.
- Social skill training.

11.13 NON-ORGANIC ENURESIS

DEFINITION

- About 50% of children by the age of 2 years and 75% by the age of 3 years are dry at night.
- Bedwetting becomes a disorder only when a child is older than 5 years.
- There are two types of enuresis:
  - primary enuresis (lifelong bedwetting);
  - secondary enuresis (free of bedwetting for 6 months):
    - diurnal,
    - nocturnal.

EPIDEMIOLOGY

- 10% at age 5 years.
- 5% at age 10 years.
- 1% at age 18 years.
- 25% with psychiatric disturbance.
- Male to female ratio: 2:1.

AETIOLOGY/RISK FACTORS

- Primary enuresis:
  - genetics;
  - small bladder;
  - large family size;
  - social adversity;
  - low IQ;
  - institutional upbringing.
- Secondary enuresis:
  - stress;
  - medical illnesses such as urinary tract infection, diabetes and chronic renal failure.

CLINICAL FEATURES

- For a child aged 5–7 years, the frequency of bedwetting is more than two times per month.
- For a child older than 7 years, the frequency of bedwetting is more than once per month.
- Duration of symptoms: at least 3 months.

INVESTIGATION

- Mid-stream urine.
- Urodynamic study if the child is older than 15 years.

TREATMENT

- Fluid restriction at night.
- Behaviour therapy: using a star chart or stickers to reward the child for dryness. This is effective in one-third of children with enuresis.
- Alarm to remind the child to wake up and urinate. It takes 8 weeks to produce dryness and is effective in 70 90% of cases.
- Medication: tricyclic antidepressants or desmopressin (an antidiuretic hormone analogue), which is reserved for severe cases.

11.14 ADOLESCENT DEPRESSION

EPIDEMIOLOGY

- Prevalence: 8%.
- Male to female ratio: 1:4.

AETIOLOGY/RISK FACTORS

- Adverse life events.
- Arguments with parents.
- Multiple family disadvantages.
- Positive family history of depression.

CLINICAL SYMPTOMS

- Similar to adult presentation.
- Promiscuity may be the presenting feature.
- Mean duration of illness is 7–9 months.
- Less likely to have psychomotor retardation when compared with adults.

INVESTIGATIONS

- Thyroid function test.

MANAGEMENT

> **MICRO-reference**
> http://www.nice.org.uk/nicemedia/live/10970/29856/29856.pdf

- Mild depression:
  - watchful waiting for 2 weeks;
  - supportive psychotherapy;

- group-based cognitive behavioural therapy (CBT);
- guided self-help;
- no antidepressant is required.
- Moderate to severe depression (including psychotic depression):
  - individual CBT or interpersonal therapy;
  - short-term family therapy;
  - if the adolescent does not respond, consider alternative psychotherapy or add fluoxetine after MDT review.
- Use of antidepressants:
  - fluoxetine 10 mg/day is the first-line treatment for those who need antidepressants;
  - citalopram and sertraline can be also used;
  - antidepressants should be discontinued slowly over 6–12 weeks to reduce discontinuation symptoms;
  - avoid tricyclic antidepressants (TCAs), paroxetine, venlafaxine and St John's wort.

PROGNOSIS

- Recurrence rate: 40% by 2 years.
- Conversion to bipolar disorder: 40% by 2 years.

11.15 ADOLESCENT SUICIDE AND DELIBERATE SELF-HARM

EPIDEMIOLOGY

- Deliberate self-harm is common among adolescents.
- Female to male ratio for deliberate self-harm: 6:1.
- Suicide is the third most common cause of death after accident and homicide in young people.
- Suicide is commonest among adolescents who are 14–16 years.
- Male to male ratio for suicide: 4:1.

AETIOLOGY/RISK FACTORS

- Depression.
- Psychosis.
- Substance misuse.
- Emotional instability.
- CD.
- Isolation.
- Low self-esteem.

- Physical illness.
- Loss of parents in childhood.
- Family dysfunction, abuse and neglect.
- Parental divorce.
- Copy-cat phenomenon: fostering of illusions and ideals through internet suicide groups and pop culture.
- Bullying in school.
- Guilt associated with abortion after teenage pregnancy.

CLINICAL RISK FACTORS

- Cutting or self-laceration is a common deliberate self-harm method.
- Self-poisoning is a common suicide method.

MANAGEMENT

- Self-laceration:
  - offer physical treatment with adequate analgesics;
  - offer psychosocial assessment and explain the care process;
  - treat underlying condition (e.g. depression);
  - alternative coping strategies to avoid self-harm.
- High suicide risk:
  - consider inpatient treatment if patient has high suicide risk;
  - treat underlying condition (e.g. depression).

PROGNOSIS

- 10% of those who self-harm for the first time will self-harm again within 1 year.
- 4% of girls and 10% of boys will commit suicide in 5 years after the first episode of self-harm.

11.16 ADOLESCENT SUBSTANCE MISUSE

EPIDEMIOLOGY

- Two-thirds of 15- to 16-year-old adolescents smoke.
- 50% of 16- to 19-year-old adolescents are regular drinkers.
- 20% of adolescents sniff glues or solvents.
- 10% of adolescents use cannabis or amphetamine on a daily basis.

AETIOLOGY/RISK FACTORS

- Environmental factors (e.g. wide-spread drug availability, high crime rate, poverty, cultural acceptance of drugs).
- School factors (e.g. peer rejection and school failure).

- Family factors (e.g. parental substance misuse and family conflict).
- Individual risk factors (e.g. low self-esteem, high sensation seeking and self-destruction).

MANAGEMENT

- Refer to substance misuse service for young people.
- Enhance collaboration between school and other agencies.
- Harm reduction (e.g. needle exchange programme).
- Motivational enhancement to quit substances.
- Family therapy.

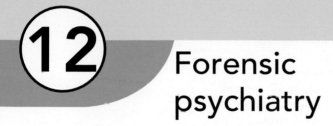

12 Forensic psychiatry

12.1 ASSESSMENT

- Psychiatrists assess patients in a variety of settings:
  - secure hospitals;
  - prisons;
  - police stations;
  - psychiatric wards.
- Other considerations:
  - try to obtain the patient's medical records from the general practitioner (GP);
  - liaise with any involved mental health teams;
  - obtain details of the current offence and any previous offences;
  - does the patient need to be treated in a psychiatric unit?
- Questions that the forensic psychiatrist has to try to answer:
  - Does this patient have a mental disorder?
  - What is the connection between the mental disorder and the offence?
  - How will treatment affect the likelihood of any future offences?
  - Does the patient require detention in a psychiatric unit?
  - Will their current mental health impact on their ability to attend court?

> **MICRO-facts**
>
> A thorough risk assessment is an integral part of the forensic psychiatrist's assessment. See Chapter 1 History and mental state examination, Risk assessment on how to complete a comprehensive risk assessment.

12.2 CRIME AND MENTAL HEALTH

> **MICRO-print**
> Approximately 5% of people who have committed homicide have schizophrenia, compared with just 1% in the general population.

SCHIZOPHRENIA

- Often commit minor offences:
  - shop lifting;
  - damage to property.
- Violence is rare and usually domestic.
- Schizophrenia and homicide:
  - associated factors include:
    - young age,
    - male gender,
    - substance abuse;
  - often secondary to severe psychosis after poor treatment compliance;
  - these patients are more likely to be victims than offenders.

MOOD DISORDER

- Minor 'out-of-character' offences:
  - shop-lifting.
- Homicide is rare:
  - usually infanticide related to a delusional belief that the victim is terminally ill (e.g. post-natal depression);
  - often followed by suicide.
- Offences linked to mania include:
  - fraud;
  - defaulted debt.

PERSONALITY DISORDERS

- Greater association with crime than any other mental disorder.
- Aspects of personality disorders related to crime include:
  - lack of empathy;
  - impulsive behaviour;
  - disturbed relationships;
  - poor anger control;
  - unstable emotions;
  - histrionic traits.

ALCOHOL AND SUBSTANCE MISUSE

- Associated with many crimes:
  - theft;
  - robbery;
  - assault;
  - homicide.

- When acutely intoxicated:
    - can lead to driving offences.
- Alcohol associated with morbid or pathological jealousy:
    - homicide of spouse.

DEMENTIA

- Occasionally shoplifting.
- Sexual offences.

12.3 LEGAL COMPETENCE

FITNESS TO PLEAD

- In order to be fit to plead the defendant requires:
    - understanding of:
        - nature of charges,
        - meaning of guilty and not guilty plea;
    - capacity to:
        - instruct solicitors,
        - challenge jurors,
        - follow court proceedings/evidence.

INSANITY DEFENCE

- Not guilty by reason of insanity.
- McNaughton criteria must be met.
- Usually used in acutely psychotic patients.

MICRO-print
McNaughton criteria
At the time of committing the act the defendant:

- had a defect of reason from disease of the mind;
- was unaware of the nature and quality of the act;
- if aware, did not know that the act was wrong.

DIMINISHED RESPONSIBILITY

- Reduces the charge of murder to manslaughter.
- Based on a specific mental disorder.
- Impaired mental responsibility owing to mental illness.

Mental health disorders

13.1 ANTIDEPRESSANTS

The mechanism of action of antidepressant agents is illustrated in (Fig. 13.1).

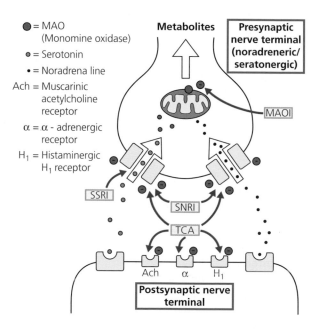

Fig. 13.1 Mechanism of action of antidepressant agents at the level of the synapse. α, alpha-adrenergic receptor; Ach, muscarinic acetylcholine receptor; H_1, histaminergic H_1 receptor; MAOI, monoamine oxidase inhibitor; TCA, tricyclic antidepressant; SNRI, serotonin–noradrenaline re-uptake inhibitor; SSRI, selective serotonin re-uptake inhibitor.

USE OF ANTIDEPRESSANTS

- Only use antidepressants in moderate to severe depression.
- Response rate in moderate to severe depression:
  - 50% response to an antidepressant;

- 30% response to placebo;
- 20% regression without treatment.
- Onset of therapeutic response:
  - within 1 week of starting;
  - response rate peaks in weeks 1–2;
  - response rate lowest in weeks 4–6.
- Starting antidepressants:
  - **first line** – selective serotonin re-uptake inhibitor (SSRI);

MICRO-facts

In patients under 18 years avoid the use of paroxetine as it can increase suicidality in this age group. Fluoxetine is the only SSRI supported by the National Institute for Health and Clinical Excellence (NICE) for use in children and adolescents. Remember that psychological interventions should be used as a first line.

  - titrate drug according to clinical response;
  - monitor all patients recently started on antidepressants closely for increased agitation and suicidal behaviour, especially if younger than 30 years;
  - if no response to drug after 2 weeks at therapeutic dose assess weekly for a further 2 weeks then consider increasing dose;
  - if side-effects are unacceptable to the patient switch to a different drug, titrate to a therapeutic dose and assess over 4 weeks;
  - if response to drug is good then maintain dose for a minimum of 6–9 months after condition improves.
- Switching antidepressants:
  - **first line** – an alternative SSRI;
  - **second line** – an antidepressant from a different class;
  - consider the half-life of the drug(s) used before switching (e.g. fluoxetine has a long half-life therefore you may need to wait before starting a different drug).
- Stopping antidepressants:
  - gradually reduce the dose over 4 weeks, except:
    - fluoxetine – not necessary because of long half-life,
    - paroxetine and venlafaxine – need to discontinue over a longer period of time;
  - discontinuation symptoms are common, although usually mild and self-limiting:
    - mood change,
    - sweating,
    - dizziness,

Mental health disorders

- insomnia,
- anxiety,
- nausea,
- flu-like symptoms.

> **MICRO-reference**
>
> National Institute for Health and Clinical Excellence. *Depression in adults.*
> *CG90.* London: National Institute for Health and Clinical Excellence, 2009.

SELECTIVE SEROTONIN RE-UPTAKE INHIBITORS

- Examples:
  - fluoxetine, paroxetine, citalopram, sertraline (e.g. fluoxetine 20 mg once daily increased after 3–4 weeks to maximum dose of 60 mg once daily if necessary).
- Mechanism of action:
  - selectively blocks re-uptake of serotonin (5-hydroxytryptamine, 5-HT) at presynaptic nerve terminals, therefore increasing synaptic serotonin concentrations.
- Indications:
  - depressive illness;
  - anxiety disorders;
  - obsessive–compulsive disorder;
  - bulimia nervosa (use fluoxetine).
- Contraindications:
  - mania.
- Side-effects:
  - gastrointestinal (GI) disturbance (nausea, vomiting, dyspepsia, abdominal pain, diarrhoea, constipation);
  - anorexia;
  - weight loss;
  - hypersensitivity reactions;
  - insomnia;
  - agitation;
  - tremor;
  - sexual dysfunction.
- Other information:
  - less sedating than tricyclic antidepressants (TCAs) therefore better tolerated;
  - may increase suicidality, therefore close monitoring of patients (especially at initiation) is important;
  - monitoring is particularly important in children and adolescents;

- dose is titrated according to clinical response:
  - the maintenance dose is the dose at which maximum benefit (symptom resolution) combined with minimum side-effects is achieved.

TRICYCLIC ANTIDEPRESSANTS

- Examples:
  - amitriptyline, nortriptyline, imipramine, clomipramine, trazodone (e.g. amitriptyline 75 mg at night increased gradually to 150–200 mg if necessary).
- Mechanism of action:
  - blocks presynaptic re-uptake of both serotonin and noradrenaline, therefore increasing synaptic neurotransmitter concentrations;
  - also block histaminergic H_1, alpha-adrenergic and cholinergic muscarinic receptors on the postsynaptic membrane.
- Indications:
  - depressive illness;
  - anxiety disorders;
  - nocturnal enuresis (use amitriptyline, nortriptyline, imipramine);
  - neuropathic pain (use amitriptyline, nortriptyline);
  - migraine prophylaxis (use amitriptyline).
- Contraindications:
  - immediately post-myocardial infarction;
  - arrhythmias;
  - epilepsy;
  - prostatic hypertrophy;
  - mania;
  - severe liver disease.
- Side-effects (Table 13.1).

Table 13.1 Side-effects of tricyclic antidepressants.

	SIDE-EFFECTS
Anticholinergic	Constipation, blurred vision, urinary retention, dry mouth
Alpha-adrenergic	Dizziness, syncope, postural hypotension
Cardiac	Arrhythmias, ECG changes (QT prolongation), tachycardia, heart block
Others	Nausea, vomiting, weight gain (from histaminergic and dopaminergic blockade), sedation, sexual dysfunction, hyponatraemia (especially elderly patients)

ECG, electrocardiogram.

Mental health disorders

- Other information:
  - extremely cardiotoxic in overdose therefore avoid in patients with risk of suicide.

MICRO-facts

Serotonin syndrome is an acute toxic syndrome caused by high levels of serotonin (e.g. concurrent use of TCAs and SSRIs). Features of serotonin syndrome are:

- confusion;
- hallucinations;
- agitation;
- headache;
- sweating;
- tachycardia;
- hypertension;
- nausea and vomiting;
- myoclonus;
- tremor;
- hyper-reflexia.

MONOAMINE OXIDASE INHIBITORS

- Examples of monoamine oxidase inhibitors (MAOIs):
  - phenelzine, isocarboxazid, tranylcypromine (e.g. phenelzine 15 mg three times a day increased after 2 weeks to 4 times a day if necessary).
- Mechanism of action:
  - inhibit the mitochondrial enzyme monoamine oxidase (MAO);
  - MAO breaks down presynaptic monoamines;
  - inhibition of MAO therefore leads to an increase in the levels of serotonin, noradrenaline, adrenaline, dopamine and tyramine available for neurotransmission;
  - MAO enzymes are found in the central nervous system (CNS), the sympathetic nervous system, the liver and the GI tract therefore inhibition of these enzymes occurs across all systems.
- Indications:
  - depressive illness.
- Contraindications:
  - liver disease;
  - phaeochromocytoma;
  - cerebrovascular disease;

- mania;
  - hyperthyroidism (tranylcypromine).
- Side-effects:
  - similar to TCAs.
- Other information:
  - need to use extreme caution when switching antidepressants to/from MAOIs;
  - inhibition of gut MAO enzyme A necessitates a low tyramine diet in these patients to avoid potentially fatal hypertensive crisis;
  - foods to be avoided:
    - mature cheese (e.g. cheddar, stilton, mozzarella),
    - cured meats (e.g. salami and pâté),
    - Marmite,
    - certain alcohols (e.g. liqueurs),
    - stale food.

OTHER ANTIDEPRESSANTS

Features of other antidepressant agents are listed in Table 13.2

> **MICRO-reference**
>
> Joint Formulary Committee. *British National Formulary*, 61st edn. London: British Medical Association and Royal Pharmaceutical Society, 2011.

13.2 ANTIPSYCHOTICS

GENERAL INFORMATION

- Typical antipsychotics are only effective against positive psychotic symptoms (e.g. hallucinations).
- Antipsychotics can take up to 2 weeks to relieve psychotic symptoms.
- Rapid tranquillization effects are immediate with, for example, haloperidol and control of mania with olanzapine.
- The half-life of antipsychotics is roughly 24 ± 9 hours (depending on drug).
- Antipsychotics have three main actions:
  - sedation;
  - tranquillization;
  - relief of psychotic symptoms.
- Efficacy in psychotic disorders:
  - $\sim 60\%$ of patients will respond to some degree;
  - $\sim 30\%$ of patients will show complete response;
  - $\sim 30\%$ of patients will show only limited improvement;

Table 13.2 Features of other antidepressant agents.

CHARACTERISTIC	MIRTAZAPINE	VENLAFAXINE	MOCLOBEMIDE
Class of drug	Noradrenergic and specific serotonergic antidepressant (NaSSA).	Serotonin–noradrenaline re-uptake inhibitor (SNRI)	Reversible inhibitor of monoamine oxidase A (RIMA)
Mechanism of action	Blocks presynaptic alpha$_2$-adrenergic receptors and postsynaptic serotonin receptors to increase synaptic serotonin and noradrenaline. Also blocks postsynaptic alpha-adrenergic, muscarinic and histaminergic receptors	Blocks re-uptake of serotonin and noradrenaline with little effect on muscarinic, histaminergic and alpha-adrenergic receptors. Also blocks re-uptake of dopamine to some extent	Reversible inhibitor of the monoamine oxidase A enzyme
Indications	Major depression. Mirtazapine causes less sexual dysfunction and is therefore indicated for patients who encounter selective serotonin re-uptake inhibitor (SSRI)-induced sexual dysfunctions	Major depression, generalized anxiety disorder	Depressive illness, social anxiety disorder
Contraindications	Breast-feeding	Arrhythmias, uncontrolled hypertension, pregnancy	Acute confusional states, phaeochromocytoma
Side-effects	Sedation, increased appetite, weight gain, dry mouth, postural hypotension, tremor, dizziness, anxiety, insomnia	Constipation, nausea, vomiting, dyspepsia, diarrhoea, anorexia, weight changes, hypertension, palpitation, pyrexia, dizziness, dry mouth, insomnia, sexual dysfunction	Sleep disturbance, dizziness, gastrointestinal symptoms, headache, agitation, paraesthesia, dry mouth, confusion, visual changes

- ~30% of patients will not respond initially, but 60% of these will go on to respond to clozapine;
- ~10% of patients will not respond to any antipsychotic agents.

MICRO-facts

Smoking, caffeine, food and antacids all alter the absorption of antipsychotics so it is important to discuss this with patients before starting them on an antipsychotic.

USE OF ANTIPSYCHOTICS

- Starting antipsychotics:
  - base choice of drug on a discussion with the patient about potential side-effects;
  - start at the lowest possible dose and titrate up;
  - in general practice, antipsychotics should only be initiated if the general practitioner (GP) has experience in treating and managing schizophrenia;
  - certain baseline tests may be needed depending on the drug being started;
  - do an electrocardiogram (ECG) if:
    - the patient is at cardiovascular risk (e.g. hypertension),
    - the patient has a past medical history of cardiovascular disease,
    - the patient is being admitted as an inpatient.
- Switching antipsychotics:
  - trial antipsychotic at maximum dose for 4–6 weeks before changing agents (if inadequate response);
  - important to check compliance if ineffective;
  - if two or more antipsychotics are ineffective at maximum dose (at least one of which is an atypical agent) then offer clozapine;
  - if unresponsive to clozapine consider augmentation with another agent that does not compound effects of clozapine;
  - augmentation should be trialed for 8–10 weeks.
- Stopping antipsychotics:
  - **first episode** – review antipsychotic use and necessity after 2 years;
  - **relapse** – need long-term antipsychotics with regular reviews.

MICRO-reference

National Institute for Health and Clinical Excellence. *Schizophrenia*. CG82. London: National Institute for Health and Clinical Excellence, 2009.

TYPICAL ANTIPSYCHOTICS

- Examples (Table 13.3)

Table 13.3 **Examples of typical antipsychotics.**

CLASS OF ANTIPSYCHOTIC	EXAMPLES
Phenothiazines – group 1 (aliphatic side-chain)	Chlorpromazine, levomepromazine
Phenothiazines – group 2 (piperidine side-chain)	Pipotiazine, pericyazine
Phenothiazines – group 3 (piperazine side-chain)	Trifluoperazine, perphenazine, prochlorpromazine
Butyrophenones	Benperidol, haloperidol
Diphenylbutylpiperidines	Pimozide
Thioxanthenes	Flupentixol, zuclopenthixol
Substituted benzamines	Sulpiride

- Mechanism of action:
    - antagonism of dopamine D_2 receptors in the entire brain;
    - clinical benefit is derived from blockade of the mesolimbic D_2 receptors;
    - antipsychotics also block muscarinic, histaminergic and alpha-adrenergic receptors to varying degrees (depending on drug in question).
- Indications:
    - schizophrenia and other psychoses;
    - mania;
    - psychomotor agitation;
    - excitement and violent/dangerously impulsive behaviour (use chlorpromazine, pericyazine, perphenazine, trifluoperazine);
    - Tourette's syndrome (use haloperidol);
    - intractable hiccup (use haloperidol);
    - nausea and vomiting in palliative care (use haloperidol, levomepromazine);
    - pain in palliative care (use levomepromazine);
    - antiemesis (use trifluoperazine, prochlorperazine).
- Contraindications:
    - Parkinson's disease (use haloperidol);
    - Lewy body dementia (use haloperidol);
    - comatose states and CNS depression;
    - phaeochromocytoma;

- pregnancy and breast-feeding:
  - use with caution,
  - antipsychotics can be given to pregnant and breast-feeding women if clinically indicated;
- excitable and overactive patients (flupentixol);
- renal impairment (pericyazine);
- agitation and restlessness in the elderly (perphenazine);
- history of arrhythmias or congenital QT prolongation (pimozide);
- acute porphyria (sulpiride);
- apathy (zuclopenthixol).
- Side-effects:
  - the major side-effects of the different antipsychotics depend on their antagonistic effects at different hormone receptors and the site of these receptors;
  - there are four main dopamine pathways in the brain (Fig. 13.2):
    - mesolimbic pathway (blockade leads to relief of psychotic symptoms),
    - mesocortical pathway,
    - nigrostriatal pathway in the basal ganglia,
    - tuberoinfundibular pathway;
  - akathisia, tardive dyskinesia, pseudoparkinsonism and acute dystonic reactions are collectively known as **extrapyramidal side-effects (EPSE)**.
  - other side-effects of antipsychotics – see Table 13.4;
  - drowsiness (histaminergic side-effect) may affect driving and use of heavy machinery;
  - each different drug and class of typical (or atypical – see below) agents has its own side-effect profile depending on the degree of blockade at different receptors:
    - chlorpromazine leads to a photosensitive blue/grey rash,
    - chlorpromazine leads to cholestatic jaundice,
    - phenothiazines and sulpiride are hepatotoxic,
    - pericyazine, sulpiride and levomepromazine are nephrotoxic,
    - promazine can lead to haemolytic anaemia,
    - pimozide can lead to QT prolongation,
    - haloperidol can lead to neuroleptic malignant syndrome,
    - chlorpromazine can lead to hyperglycaemia;
  - it is important to discuss the full side-effects of each drug with the patient before starting and tailor it to the individual;
  - phenothiazines have different predominating side-effects depending on their side-chain (Table 13.5);
  - all of the other typical agents have side-effects resembling those of the antipsychotics with a piperazine side-chain.

Mental health disorders

Mental health disorders

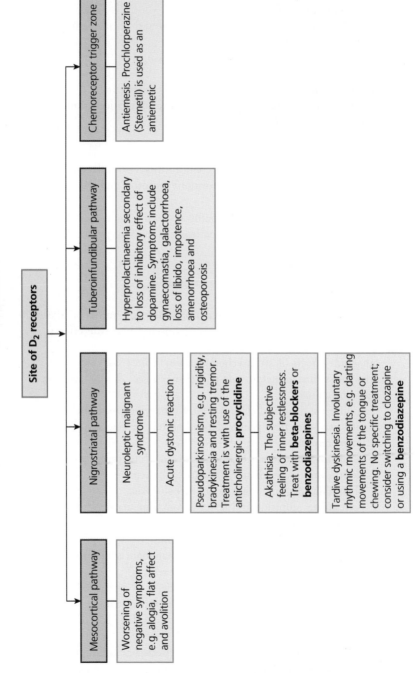

Fig. 13.2 Dopaminergic side-effects of antipsychotics.

Table 13.4 Other side-effects of antipsychotics.

Anticholinergic	Dry mouth, blurred vision, angle closure glaucoma (rare), urinary retention, urinary hesitancy, constipation, tachycardia, confusion
Anti-adrenergic	Dizziness, postural hypotension, impotence
Histaminergic	Weight gain, sedation
Cardiac	Prolongation of QT, which can lead to ventricular tachyarrhythmias (e.g. torsades de pointes) leading to sudden death
Others	Blood dyscrasias, photosensitivity, cholestatic jaundice, pancytopenia, agranulocytosis, decreased seizure threshold, venous thromboembolism, corneal and lens opacities

Table 13.5 Relative side-effects of the different classes of phenothiazine antipsychotics.

	DOPAMINERGIC EPSE	ANTI-CHOLINERGIC SIDE-EFFECTS	HISTAMINERGIC SIDE-EFFECTS
Aliphatic side-chain (e.g. chlorpromazine)	+ +	+ +	+ + +
Piperidine side-chain (e.g. pipotiazine)	+	+ + +	+ +
Piperazine side-chain (e.g. trifluoperazine)	+ + +	+	+

EPSE, extrapyramidal side-effects.

ATYPICAL ANTIPSYCHOTICS

- Examples:
  - amisulpride, clozapine, risperidone, olanzapine, zotepine and quetiapine.
- Mechanism of action:
  - block dopamine D_2 receptors in the whole brain as well as histaminergic, acetylcholine and α-adrenergic receptors to varying degrees;
  - block serotonin $5HT_{2A}$ receptors.

Mental health disorders

- Indications and contraindications:
  - as for typical antipsychotics (see Typical antipsychotics, above).
- Side-effects:
  - unlike typical agents, atypical antipsychotics have a relatively low affinity for nigrostriatal D_2 dopamine receptors, therefore EPSEs are much less common making them much better tolerated;
  - other side-effects are similar to those of typical agents (see Typical antipsychotics, above);
  - some important drug-specific side-effects are:
    - clozapine:
      - ○ agranulocytosis – can be fatal so monitor full blood count (FBC),

---

MICRO-facts

Monitoring of FBC with clozapine:

- before commencing clozapine;
- every 1 week for 18 weeks;
- every 2 weeks for rest of first year;
- every 4 weeks from then on.

It is important to register patients on clozapine with the **clozapine patient monitoring service**.

      - ○ myocarditis and cardiomyopathy,
      - ○ intestinal obstruction,
      - ○ hypersalivation,
      - ○ risk of seizures;
    - risperidone:
      - ○ hyperprolactinaemia,
      - ○ EPSE can occur at high doses;
    - olanzapine:
      - ○ weight gain,
      - ○ high risk of diabetes,
      - ○ anticholinergic side-effects;
    - quetiapine:
      - ○ alpha-adrenergic side-effects,
      - ○ weight gain.

NEWER ANTIPSYCHOTICS

- Example:
  - aripiprazole.
- Mechanism of action:
  - partial agonism at D_2 and $5-HT_{1A}$ receptors;

- antagonism at $5HT_{2A}$ receptors;
- moderate affinity for D_4, $5HT_{2C}$, $5HT_7$, adrenergic, and histaminergic receptors.
- Indications and contraindications:
  - as for typical antipsychotics (see Typical antipsychotics, above).
- Side-effects:
  - headache;
  - insomnia;
  - agitation;
  - anxiety.

ANTIPSYCHOTIC DEPOT INJECTIONS

- Examples:
  - fluphenazine decanoate 12.5–100 mg every 2–5 weeks;
  - haloperidol 50–300 mg every 4 weeks;
  - risperidone 25–50 mg every 2 weeks;
  - olanzapine embonate 150–300 mg every 2–4 weeks;
  - pipotiazine palmitate 50–200 mg every 4 weeks.
- Indications:
  - NICE recommends the use of this preparation of antipsychotic if:
    - the patient prefers a depot to oral medication,
    - non-compliance to oral medication is an issue.
- Limitations:
  - if side-effects occur it can take some weeks for the drug effects to wear off;
  - treatment needs careful monitoring of side-effects and therapeutic effect;
  - gradual reduction of oral dose needs to take place if changing from oral preparation.
- Choice:
  - depends on outcome of discussion with patient about potential side-effects;
  - in general, if the patient has responded to the oral preparation of the antipsychotic then this is the drug of choice;
  - zuclopenthixol is suitable for use in agitated or aggressive patients;
  - important to use small doses initially and monitor side-effects.
- Side-effects:
  - same as for oral preparation of drug (see Atypical antipsychotics, above);
  - injection site reactions may occur (e.g. pain, erythema, swelling or nodules).

13.3 MOOD STABILIZERS

INDICATIONS

- Treating acute mania (lithium and semi-sodium valproate).
- Prophylaxis in bipolar disorder.
- Refractory depression.
- Disorders with recurrent aggression or self-harming behaviour.

> **MICRO-facts**
>
> Carbamazepine and valproic acid are antiepileptic drugs also commonly used as mood stabilizers.

COMMON MOOD STABILIZERS

- Lithium is the most commonly used mood stabilizer.
- Carbamazepine.
- Valproic acid.
- Lamotrigine.

STARTING MOOD STABILIZERS

- Pre-treatment investigations:
  - lithium:
    - weight,
    - medication review:
      - ○ non-steroidal anti-inflammatory drugs (NSAIDs) and angiotensin-converting enzyme (ACE) inhibitors interact;
    - blood tests:
      - ○ FBC,
      - ○ urea and electrolytes (U&E) and estimated glomerular filtration rate (eGFR),
      - ○ thyroid function tests (TFTs),
    - electrocardiogram (ECG);
  - carbamazepine:
    - weight,
    - blood tests:
      - ○ FBC,
      - ○ liver function tests (LFTs),
      - ○ U&E;
    - ECG;

> **MICRO-facts**
>
> Be aware that the combined oral contraceptive pill (COCP) is contra-indicated in combination with some antiepileptic drugs.

- valproic acid:
  - baseline weight,
  - FBC,
  - LFTs.
- For women of childbearing age:
  - a pregnancy test is indicated before treatment with mood stabilizers as they are all teratogenic;
  - while on treatment women must therefore be advised about appropriate contraception.

CHARACTERISTICS OF MOOD STABILIZERS

- For characteristics of mood stabilizers see Table 13.6.

MECHANISM OF ACTION

- Lithium:
  - increases $Na^+/K^+/ATP$-ase activity in patients (but not in healthy individuals);
  - lithium affects the following neurotransmitters:
    - 5HT (increased synthesis and release),
    - noradrenaline (increased uptake),
    - dopamine,
    - acetylcholine (increased levels of choline);
  - also interferes with cyclic (c) AMP (inhibits Na^+-induced cAMP activity) which can lead to thyroid and kidney side-effects.

> **MICRO-facts**
>
> - Dehydration and diuretics can lead to lithium toxicity.
> - Other drugs that can interact with lithium:
>   - NSAIDs;
>   - some antibiotics;
>   - calcium channel blockers.

SIDE-EFFECTS AND CONTRAINDICATIONS

- Lithium:
  - side-effects:
    - nausea,
    - fine tremor,

Mental health disorders

Pharmacotherapy

Table 13.6 Characteristics of mood stabilizers.

CHARACTERISTIC	LITHIUM	CARBAMAZEPINE	VALPROIC ACID	LAMOTRIGINE
Mode of administration	Oral	Oral	Oral	Oral
Dose	Start at 400 mg at night Maximum 1.2–1.8 g daily Titrate to a serum lithium concentration of 0.4–1 mmol/L	400–600 mg daily Maximum dose 1.6 g daily	Initially 750 mg daily Usually 1–2 g daily	25 mg for 14 days then 50 mg for 14 days Then increase by 50–100 mg every 7–14 days 100–200 mg usual daily dose
Additional prescribing notes	Narrow therapeutic range >0.4–1.0 mmol/L Toxic >1.5 mmol/L Measure levels 12 hours after dose on day 7 Measure levels every week until levels have remained constant for 4 weeks Measure levels every 3 months thereafter Regular monitoring of FBC, U&E, Ca and TFTs	Regular monitoring of FBC	LFTs should be monitored regularly	Monitor LFTs, renal and clotting levels

FBC, full blood count; LFTs, liver function tests; TFTs, thyroid function tests; U&E, urea and electrolytes.

- weight gain,
- oedema,
- polydipsia,
- polyuria,
- hypothyroidism;
  - contraindications:
    - renal disease,
    - cardiac disease,
    - thyroid disease,
    - Addison's disease,
    - pregnancy and breast-feeding.
- Carbamazepine:
  - side-effects:
    - blood dyscrasias,
    - rashes,
    - interacts with other medications that are metabolized by the same cytochrome P450 pathway;
  - contraindications:
    - pregnancy and breast-feeding (teratogenic),
    - interferes with the oral contraceptive pill.
- Valproic acid:
  - side-effects:
    - nausea,
    - gastric irritation,
    - diarrhoea,
    - weight gain,
    - thrombocytopenia.
- Lamotrigine:
  - side-effects:
    - nausea,
    - dizziness,
    - headache,
    - diplopia,
    - nausea,
    - ataxia,
    - Steven–Johnson syndrome.

13.4 ANXIOLYTICS AND HYPNOTICS

BENZODIAZEPINES

- Examples:
  - short-acting: midazolam [half life ($t_{1/2}$) up to 12 hours];

- medium-acting: lorazepam and clonazepam ($t_{1/2}$ up to 40 hours);
- long-acting: diazepam and chlordiazepoxide ($t_{1/2} > 40$ hours).
- Mechanism of action:
  - act at the gamma-aminobutyric acid (GABA)$_A$–benzodiazepine receptor complex;
  - increase the effectiveness of GABA at its receptor by increasing Cl$^-$ entry into neurons;
  - GABA has inhibitory effects on the CNS and decreases excitability;
  - full agonism at the benzodiazepine receptor leads to sedation, reduction in anxiety (anxiolytic effect) and reduced likelihood of seizures (anticonvulsant effect).
- Indications:
  - insomnia, short-term relief;
  - severe anxiety, short-term relief;
  - alcohol withdrawal.
- Contraindications:
  - should be avoided in patients with compromised respiratory function (e.g. obstructive sleep apnoea, myasthenia gravis).
- Side-effects:
  - dependence;
  - withdrawal symptoms (increased anxiety, worsened sleep disturbance);
  - confusion;
  - amnesia;
  - ataxia;
  - may affect driving owing to sedation.

MICRO-facts

Approximate equivalent dose to 5 mg diazepam:

lorazepam = 500 micrograms;
temazepam = 10 mg;
nitrazepam = 5 mg;
chlordiazepoxide = 15 mg.

- Starting benzodiazepines:
  - insomnia:
    - start on lowest dose taken at bedtime e.g. nitrazepam 5 mg,
    - increase if needed,
    - short-term use of up to 2 weeks;
  - anxiety:
    - start on lowest dose taken in three divided doses (e.g. diazepam 2 mg three times a day),

- – increase if not effective,
- – short-term use only.
- Stopping benzodiazepines:
  - step-down gradually especially if prolonged use;
  - decrease dose by one-eighth per fortnight;
  - if experiencing withdrawal symptoms remain on dose until subsided.

NON-BENZODIAZEPINE HYPNOTICS

- Examples:
  - zopiclone, zolpidem, zaleplon (z-drugs).
- Mechanism of action:
  - also act on the $GABA_A$–benzodiazepine receptor complex to increase GABA action and therefore inhibit neuronal activity.
- Indications:
  - insomnia.
- Contraindications:
  - obstructive sleep apnoea.
- Side-effects:
  - amnesia;
  - drowsiness;
  - taste disturbance.
- Starting non-benzodiazepine hypnotics:
  - taken at bedtime (e.g. zopiclone 7.5 mg);
  - prescribe at lowest dose and increase if needed.

BUSPIRONE

- Mechanism of action:
  - buspirone is an SSRI (see the section on Antidepressants above).
- Indications:
  - short-term anxiety.
- Side-effects:
  - nausea;
  - dizziness;
  - headache.
- Starting buspirone:
  - 5 mg two or three times daily;
  - usual dose 15–30 mg per day in divided doses;
  - maximum dose 45 mg.

PRESCRIBING ANXIOLYTICS AND HYPNOTICS

- Short term insomnia:
  - prescribe a benzodiazepine or z-drug:
    - temazepam, loprazolam, lormetazepam,
    - zopiclone, zolpidem, zaleplon;
  - prescribe at the lowest effective dose;
  - if one z-drug is ineffective do not try another.

MICRO-facts

For patients who have difficulty getting to sleep:

- short-acting hypnotics are best;
- tolerance and dependence can develop fast.

For patients with frequent early morning waking:

- longer-acting drugs are best;
- next day sedation (hangover effect) is more likely.

- Generalized anxiety disorder:
  - first-line treatment is an SSRI (see the section on Antidepressants above):
    - escitalopram, paroxetine;
  - do not prescribe benzodiazepines for more than 2 weeks.
- Panic disorder:
  - first-line treatment is an SSRI (see the section on Antidepressants above):
    - citalopram, escitalopram, paroxetine;
  - do not routinely prescribe benzodiazepines.

14 Electroconvulsive therapy and psychotherapy

14.1 ELECTROCONVULSIVE THERAPY

> **MICRO-facts**
>
> Before using electroconvulsive therapy (ECT) other treatments must have failed and/or the condition must have become life threatening (e.g. refusal of food and drink or suicide risk).

INDICATIONS

- Severe depressive illness.
- Severe mania.
- Catatonia.

MECHANISM OF ACTION

- Induces a generalized tonic–clonic seizure.
- Consecutive treatments induce:
  - neurotransmitter release;
  - increase in permeability of the blood–brain barrier;
  - release of hypothalamic and pituitary hormones;
  - modulation of neurotransmitter receptors.

PROCEDURE

The electroconvulsive therapy (ECT) procedural pathway is illustrated in Fig. 14.1.

LEGAL REQUIREMENTS

- Requires consent of patients with capacity.
- Cannot be given to a patient with capacity who does not consent.
- A second opinion is required for patients aged under 18 years.
- A second opinion is needed if the patient lacks capacity (unable to consent) or in cases of detained patients who refuse to consent.

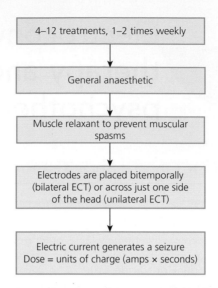

Fig. 14.1 Electroconvulsive therapy (ECT) procedural pathway.

- Exceptionally, ECT can be given without consent if given as an urgent life-saving treatment.

CONTRAINDICATIONS

- No absolute contraindications.
- Relative contraindications:
    - raised intracranial pressure;
    - recent stroke;
    - recent myocardial infarction;
    - crescendo angina.

SIDE-EFFECTS

- Headache.
- Muscle pain.
- Drowsiness.
- Loss of recent memories (retrograde amnesia).
- Anterograde amnesia (less common than retrograde amnesia):
    - may persist for several weeks;
    - may be reduced by unilateral electrode placement.
- Confusion.
- Prolonged seizures.

COMPLICATIONS

- Anaesthetic complications.
- Dysrhythmias.
- Pulmonary embolism (PE), aspiration pneumonia and cerebrovascular accidents (CVAs).
- Factors associated with an increase in seizure threshold:
    - old age;
    - male gender;
    - baldness;
    - Paget's disease;
    - dehydration;
    - previous ECT;
    - benzodiazepine treatment.
- Factors associated with a reduction in seizure threshold:
    - caffeine;
    - low CO_2 saturation of blood;
    - hyperventilation;
    - theophylline.

14.2 PSYCHOTHERAPY

COGNITIVE BEHAVIOURAL THERAPY

- Indications:
    - depression;
    - eating disorders;
    - anxiety disorders;
    - obsessive–compulsive disorder;
    - post-traumatic stress disorder;
    - chronic psychosis.
- Treatment:
    - frequency usually weekly;
    - normally 6–12 sessions.
- Cognitive methods:
    - identify negative automatic thoughts;
    - complete a thought diary to highlight connections between thoughts, emotions and behaviour;
    - examine and challenge evidence for and against negative automatic thoughts and learn to replace them with more realistic explanations.
- Behavioural methods:
    - relaxation techniques;

Mental health disorders

- desensitization:
  - hierarchy of anxiety-provoking situations,
  - exposed to them gradually;
- flooding (very rarely used):
  - exposure to the phobic object without prior reduction in anxiety,
  - continue with the exposure until the anxiety is reduced;
- schedule of activities (used in those with poor motivation).

PSYCHODYNAMIC PSYCHOTHERAPY

- Indications:
  - personality disorders;
  - psychosexual problems;
  - somatoform disorders;
  - recurrent depression.
- Treatment:
  - usually one or two sessions a week;
  - the total number of sessions is variable.
- What it involves:
  - discussing past experiences and how they have shaped the current situation;
  - exploring unconscious thoughts;
  - aim to relieve symptoms and modify personalities;
  - great emphasis on the relationship between the therapist and the patient;
  - therapy can be individual, couple or group.

INTERPERSONAL PSYCHOTHERAPY

- Indications:
  - depression (non-psychotic);
  - eating disorders.
- Treatment:
  - weekly sessions;
  - normally 12–20 sessions in total.
- What it involves:
  - focuses on interpersonal aspects of the illness;
  - careful discussion of close relationships;
  - any problems highlighted are conceptualized and are discussed in future sessions;
  - links between symptoms and interpersonal problems examined.

OTHER PSYCHOTHERAPIES

- Some other therapies worth noting:
  - dialectical behaviour therapy (see Chapter 10 Disorders of adult personality, Treatment);
  - family therapy;
  - group therapy;
  - supportive therapies (counselling).

15 Psychiatric emergencies

15.1 SUICIDE

EPIDEMIOLOGY

- Male to female ratio: 3:1.
- Incidence increases with increasing age.
- In the UK there are around 5000 suicides a year and around 140 000 attendances for attempted suicide.

> **MICRO-print**
> Since 2002 the UK has had a suicide prevention strategy and deaths from suicides have fallen to 7.8 per 100,000.
> More details and resources may be found at http://www.nmhdu.org.uk

AETIOLOGY

- Risk factors:
  - male;
  - older age;
  - single/divorced;
  - previous suicide attempt;
  - mental illness (depression or psychosis);
  - alcohol/drug abuse (see Chapter 5 Substance misuse);
  - isolation/lack of social network;
  - professions (farmer, doctor, dentist, vet);
  - chronic illness;
  - significant life event (e.g. death, losing job, relationship breakdown, abuse).

SCREENING QUESTIONS

- Routine screening:
  - Have you thought about harming yourself?
  - Have you thought about taking your own life?

- What has stopped you so far?
- Do you think you would act on these thoughts?
- Have you made any plans?
- General questions:
  - Was it planned?
  - What was the intent?
  - Was anyone else there/were you likely to be found?
  - Was a note left?
  - How did you come to be in the emergency department (ED)?
  - How do you feel about it now (regret)?
  - Would you do it again?
  - How do you feel about the future?
  - Have you attempted suicide previously?
  - Do you have a history of mental illness?
  - Are you suffering from any other illnesses?
  - Has anything changed in your life recently (for example, death of spouse)?
  - Events leading up to the attempt?
  - Take a depression history (see Chapter 7 Affective disorders, Depressive episode).
  - Take a psychosis history (see Chapter 6 Schizophrenia and delusional disorders, Schizophrenia).
  - Take a general history (see Chapter 1 History and mental state examination, Psychiatric history).

MICRO-facts

Mnemonic for assessment of risk:

Sex = male	1
Age <19 years or > 45 years	1
Depressed/hopeless	2
Previous suicide attempts	1
Excessive alcohol/drug use	1
Rational thinking loss (psychosis)	2
Separated/widowed/divorced	1
Organized or serious attempt	2
No social support	1
State future intent	2

Score: < 6 = **may be safe to discharge**
          6–8 = **psychiatric assessment**
          > 8 = **urgent admission**

> **Micro-reference**
> SADPERSONS mneumonic, developed by Patterson WM, Dohn HH, Bird J, Patterson GA, *Psychosomatics* 1983; **24**: 343–9.

- Overdose:
  - What was taken?
  - How much was taken?
  - How did you get hold of the substance?
  - Taken all at once or over a period of time?
  - Was alcohol taken as well?
  - What did the patient think would happen when they took the substances?

INVESTIGATIONS

- Follow ABC (Airway, Breathing, Circulation) approach for assessment.
- If overdose:
  - bloods:
    - full blood count (FBC),
    - clotting screen,
    - liver function tests (LFTs),
    - paracetamol levels,
    - salicylate levels,
    - urea and electrolytes (U&E),
    - glucose.
- Psychiatric assessment.
- May need to find previous and third-person history from e.g. general practitioner (GP) or relatives.

MANAGEMENT

- Assess patient's risk to self, including how likely they are to attempt suicide again.
- It is highly desirable for all patients who have attempted suicide to be seen by psychiatric services before leaving hospital.

MICRO-facts

Paracetamol overdose management:

- Patients are at risk of developing acute liver failure.
- Blood sample for paracetamol levels taken 4 hours after ingestion.
- If after 4 hours, take as soon as possible.

continued...

continued...

- Level needs to be plotted on a paracetamol treatment graph.
- If treatment indicated *N*-acetylcysteine should be started; see *British National Formulary* (BNF) for doses.
- High-risk line is used for patients who are malnourished, human immunodeficiency virus (HIV)-positive, alcoholics, on anti-epileptics and have eating disorders.

MICRO-reference

Joint Formulary Committee. *British National Formulary*, 61st edn. London: British Medical Association and Royal Pharmaceutical Society, 2011.

15.2 SELF-HARM

EPIDEMIOLOGY

- Male to female ratio: male < female.
- Age of onset: most common in adolescents.
- It is estimated that 7–14% of adolescents have self-harmed (NHS UK).

MICRO-reference

http://www.nhs.uk/Conditions/Self-injury/Pages/Introduction.aspx

AETIOLOGY

- A physical expression of emotional distress:
    - grief;
    - loneliness;
    - anxiety;
    - guilt;
    - sadness.
- An expression of social problems and trauma:
    - difficult relationships with family/with a partner/with friends;
    - bullying at school or work;
    - traumatic life events, for example physical/sexual abuse, suffering a miscarriage, death of a close family member/friend;
    - problems with identity, for example sexuality, culture, gender.
- Secondary to a psychiatric disorder:
    - auditory hallucinations telling the person to harm themselves;

- compulsion to self-harm;
- part of a personality disorder.

MICRO-facts

Types of self-harm include:

- cutting, usually of arms, thighs or chest;
- burning skin;
- misusing drugs or alcohol;
- over- or under-eating.

CLINICAL FEATURES

- Physical:
    - scars;
    - bruises;
    - burns;
    - clothing to cover arms/avoidance of activities involving undressing.
- Psychological:
    - low self-esteem and self-worth;
    - depression;
    - anxiety;
    - guilt;
    - often withdrawn from family and friends.

SCREENING QUESTIONS

- When did the self-harming start?
- Was there any trigger?
- How does the person feel when they self-harm?
- What do they want to happen when they self-harm?
- How did they present to you (as a medical service)?
- How do they normally feel at the time of self-harming?
- How do they view themselves as a person (self-esteem)?
- Is there anything happening in their life at the moment that they'd like to talk about?
- How is work/school?
- Does anyone know about their self-harming?
- Do they ever think about taking the self-harm further (to suicide)?
- Take a thorough drug and alcohol history (see Chapter 5 Substance misuse, Assessment of substance misuse).

- Screen for depression and anxiety (see Chapter 7 Affective disorders, Depressive episode and Chapter 8 Anxiety and neuroses, Generalized anxiety disorder).
- Assess suicide risk.

INVESTIGATIONS

- Depending on the type of self-harm, medical assessment of injuries may be needed.
- If alcohol/drug abuse present further investigations may be relevant (e.g. abdominal ultrasound scan for liver damage; see Chapter 5 Substance misuse, Harmful use).

MICRO-print

Alternative strategies to self-harming:

- using a red marker pen instead of cutting;
- flicking an elastic band on skin;
- using an ice cube to give pain without damage.

MANAGEMENT

- Address underlying issues/cause.
- Treat depression/anxiety (see Chapter 7 Affective disorders, Depressive episode and Chapter 8 Anxiety and neuroses, Generalized anxiety disorder).
- Cognitive behavioural therapy.
- Discuss alternative coping strategies.
- Referral to drug/alcohol services.

15.3 LITHIUM TOXICITY

- Lithium is a mood stabilizer and is used in various psychiatric disorders (see Chapter 13 Pharmacotherapy, Mood stabilizers).

ADMINISTRATION AND ACTION

- It is taken orally and is excreted by the kidneys.
- Lithium has a narrow therapeutic range of 0.4–1.0 mmol/L.
- U&E, especially estimated glomerular filtration rate (eGFR) and thyroid function tests (TFTs) should be measured before starting lithium.
- TFTs should be rechecked 6-monthly.

Mental health disorders

- Careful monitoring of lithium levels and renal function should be undertaken every 3 months.
- Lithium may interact with sodium, potassium, magnesium and calcium homeostasis.

SIDE-EFFECTS

- Side-effects are dose related and include:
  - nausea;
  - fine tremor;
  - weight gain;
  - oedema;
  - polydipsia;
  - polyuria;
  - exacerbations of psoriasis and acne.

PREDISPOSING FACTORS FOR TOXICITY

- Renal failure.
- Dehydration.
- Diuretics (especially thiazides).
- Non-steroidal anti-inflammatory drugs (NSAIDs).
- Angiotensin-converting enzyme (ACE) inhibitors

TOXIC EFFECTS

- Signs of lithium levels >1.5 mmol/L:
  - vomiting;
  - diarrhoea;
  - coarse tremor;
  - slurred speech;
  - ataxia;
  - drowsiness.
- Signs of lithium levels >2.4 mmol/L:
  - increased disorientation;
  - seizures;
  - coma;
  - death.

MANAGEMENT OF TOXICITY

- Cessation of lithium.
- Serum lithium level.
- Forced diuresis (e.g. IV mannitol).
- Haemodialysis.
- Peritoneal dialysis.

15.4 NEUROLEPTIC MALIGNANT SYNDROME

EPIDEMIOLOGY

- Incidence: 0.07–0.2% of patients on antipsychotics.
- Age of onset: more common in younger patients.
- Male to female ratio: 2:1.

PATHOPHYSIOLOGY

- Excessive dopamine D_2 receptor blockade by antipsychotic leads to decreased cerebral dopamine availability.
- Frequently associated with haloperidol but can potentially occur with any antipsychotic, including atypicals.

MICRO-print

Clinical features are a reflection of the site of the dopamine blockade:

- Corpus striatum: muscle rigidity.
- Pre-optic nuclei of anterior hypothalamus (thermoregulatory centre): hyperpyrexia.
- Nigrostriatal and mesocortical systems: mental state changes.
- Spinal cord: autonomic dysfunction.

CLINICAL FEATURES

Clinical features of neuroleptic malignant syndrome (NMS) are listed in Table 15.1.

- Usually seen within 4–11 days of either starting a treatment regime or changing dose (but can be at any point during treatment course).
- Clinical features gradually evolve over 24–72 hours.
- Clinical features may last for 1–2 weeks after discontinuing oral antipsychotics, or 4–6 weeks after stopping depot antipsychotics.

INVESTIGATIONS

- Bloods:
  - FBC: shows leukocytosis;
  - LFTs: abnormal liver enzymes;
  - creatinine kinase: raised owing to rhabdomyolysis from sustained muscle contraction;
  - U&E: necessary as rhabdomyolysis can lead to renal failure.
- Vital signs:
  - raised temperature;
  - tachycardia;

Mental health disorders

Table 15.1 Clinical features of neuroleptic malignant syndrome (NMS).

Motor symptoms	Muscular hypertonicity Dystonia Akinesia Tremor
Mental signs	Fluctuating consciousness Agitation Confusion Akinetic mutism
Autonomic symptoms	Hyperpyrexia Excess sweating and salivation Tachycardia Labile blood pressure Tachypnoea Pallor Urinary incontinence

- tachypnoea;
- fluctuating blood pressure.

MANAGEMENT

- Stop antipsychotic.
- Transfer to intensive care unit (ICU).
- Supportive:
  - administer oxygen if needed;
  - cool patient down using ice packs or cold fluids;
  - if dehydrated (owing to sweating and high temperature) give IV fluids (e.g. 0.9% saline).
  - give 1 g paracetamol to reduce temperature.
- Monitor:
  - U&E to check for renal failure (secondary to rhabdomyolysis);
  - vital signs.
- Some patients may need haemodialysis.
- If agitated:
  - give a benzodiazepine (e.g. diazepam; see Chapter 13 Pharmacotherapy, Anxiolytics and hypnotics):
    - diazepam can also help with muscle stiffness.
- Dantrolene:
  - used to treat malignant hyperthermia, in NMS acts as a skeletal muscle relaxant;
  - to decrease muscle spasm.

- Bromocriptine:
  - dopamine D_2 receptor agonist and partial dopamine D_1 receptor agonist;
  - to reverse dopamine receptor blockade.

PROGNOSIS

- Mortality: 10–20% if untreated.
- Death occurs from acute renal failure secondary to rhabdomyolysis.

MICRO-case

A 23-year-old man with a known history of schizophrenia is brought onto your psychiatric inpatient ward under the Mental Health Act following a relapse. For the last 2 months he has refused to have his monthly 200 mg haloperidol depot. On admission he is given 300 mg IM haloperidol. Seven days later he is found in his bed-space sweating profusely and unable to move his arms. On examination his temperature is 38.8°C, his heart rate is 120 beats/minute with a blood pressure of 140/100 mmHg.

Learning points

- Always titrate antipsychotics up to desired dose.
- Always consider the possibility of NMS when prescribing antipsychotics.

15.5 ACUTE DYSTONIC REACTION

EPIDEMIOLOGY

- Incidence: 2%.
- Male to female ratio: male > female.
- Age of onset: decreases with age.

AETIOLOGY

- Thought to be caused by dopamine (D_2) blockade in the nigrostriatum leading to an increased cholinergic output by neuroleptic medication (e.g. haloperidol).
- Risk factors:
  - young male;
  - antipsychotic naïve;
  - use of high-dose neuroleptics;
  - history of dystonic reaction.

Mental health disorders

CLINICAL FEATURES

- Onset:
  - normally within 5 days of commencing or increasing dose of neuroleptic medication
  - sudden onset.
- Dystonic features (increase in muscle tone):
  - oculogyric crisis (rolling of eyes upwards);
  - tongue protrusion;
  - difficulty talking;
  - grimacing;
  - torticollis (twisting of neck);
  - can affect muscles of respiration.

INVESTIGATIONS

- Vital signs should be normal.
- Check drug history.
- Check mental status:
  - should be normal;
  - if not, exclude seizure.

MANAGEMENT

- Give 5 mg IM procyclidine stat.
- Add regular procyclidine (5 mg up to three times daily).
- Explain the condition to the patient and reassure.
- If patient on a typical antipsychotic, change to an atypical.

15.6 ACUTE ALCOHOL WITHDRAWAL STATE WITH DELIRIUM

EPIDEMIOLOGY

- Incidence: 5% of patients with alcohol withdrawal.
- Male to female ratio: male > female.
- Highest prevalence: young males.

AETIOLOGY

- Alcohol is a gamma-aminobutyric acid (GABA) receptor agonist and an *N*-methyl-d-aspartate (NMDA) antagonist.
- Chronic alcohol exposure reduces GABA function (leading to tolerance).
- Chronic alcohol abuse also increases NMDA receptor function:
  - leads to memory problems;
  - may provoke a hyperexcitable state with seizures in withdrawal.

- Withdrawal of alcohol leads to a lack of stimulation of GABA receptors, precipitating the clinical features of delirium tremens.

CLINICAL FEATURES

> ### MICRO-facts
>
> Delirium tremens is a medical emergency as the mortality rate is 5–15%; therefore, a high index of suspicion is necessary in patients with a history of chronic alcohol consumption and the clinical features listed in the text below.

- Onset:
  - usually 48–72 hours after cessation of drinking.
- Features of withdrawal include:
  - tremulousness;
  - agitation;
  - nausea and vomiting;
  - sweating;
  - overwhelming desire to drink.
- Features of delirium tremens include:
  - delirium;
  - visual hallucinations;
  - formication;

> ### MICRO-print
>
> Formication: a type of tactile hallucination – insects crawling under the skin.

  - delusions (persecutory);
  - fear;
  - agitation;
  - aggression;
  - coarse tremor;
  - seizures;
  - autonomic features:
    - sweating,
    - fever,
    - tachycardia,
    - hypertension;
  - insomnia;

- dehydration;
- electrolyte disturbance.

INVESTIGATIONS

- Gamma glutamyltransferase (GGT).
- Glucose: to assess for hypoglycaemia or hyperglycaemia.
- LFTs.
- International normalized ratio (INR).
- B_{12} and folate.
- FBC: macrocytic anaemia, thrombocytopenia and leucocytosis often seen.
- U&E: to assess for hyponatraemia and hypokalaemia.

> ### MICRO-facts
> The patient may have low Mg^{2+} and PO_4^{3-}.

MANAGEMENT

- Detoxification (see Fig. 15.1).

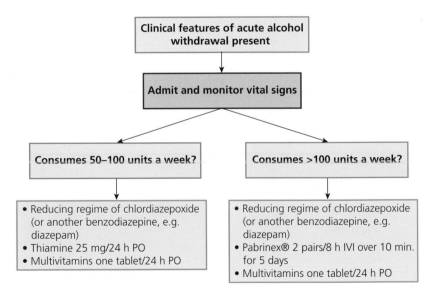

Fig. 15.1 Alcohol detoxification.

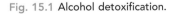

Mental health disorders

MICRO-print

- Pabrinex is given IV and is a high potency mixture of B and C vitamins.
- Chlordiazepoxide is the benzodiazepine of choice as it is long-acting and less likely to lead to dependence.
- Shorter acting benzodiazepines (e.g. lorazepam/oxazepam) should be used in patients with alcoholic liver disease, therefore it is important to check LFTs before commencing treatment.

- Reducing regime of chlordiazepoxide for moderate alcohol dependence (Table 15.2).

Table 15.2 Chlordiazepoxide doses for alcohol detoxification.

DAY	DOSE
One	20 mg orally, four times
Two	15 mg orally, four times
Three	10 mg orally, four times
Four	5 mg orally, four times
Five	5 mg orally, twice

MICRO-print

In severe dependence the initial dose may be 200–250 mg and the treatment may be extended to 10 days.

- Additional management:
  - rehydration;
  - correction of any electrolyte imbalances.

PROGNOSIS

- Mortality from delirium tremens: 5%.

15.7 AGGRESSION AND AGITATION

DEFINITION

- Any incident in which a person working in the health-care sector is verbally abused, threatened or assaulted by a patient or member of the public in circumstances relating to his or her employment.

MICRO-reference
National Institute for Health and Clinical Excellence. *Violence and aggression in general practice: guidance on assessment and management.* London: National Institute for Health and Clinical Excellence, 2001.

AETIOLOGY

- Disorders that may cause violence or aggression:
  - mental retardation;
  - attention-deficit hyperactivity disorder (ADHD);
  - conduct disorder (CD);
  - delirium;
  - dementia;
  - schizophrenia;
  - manic episode/bipolar affective disorder (BAD);
  - substance intoxication or withdrawal (including alcohol);
  - adjustment disorder;
  - paranoid, antisocial, borderline or narcissistic personality disorders (PD).

MANAGEMENT

When dealing with acutely aggressive or agitated patients, trained staff should initially try to de-escalate the situation by talking to the patient and offering them a 'time out' (i.e. moving away to a quiet area).

- Environmental assessment:
  - conduct the interview in a side-room away from the clinical environment;
  - empty the room of other patients/staff members;
  - if possible, use a room with two exits;
  - remove all potential weapons (e.g. books, chairs, telephones, etc.);
  - turn off the television/radio;
  - always have another member of staff (trained in control and restraint) present during the interview.
- Pay attention to your own behaviour:
  - stay calm;
  - place yourself closer to the exit than the patient;
  - never turn your back on the patient;
  - tell someone where you are and who you are with;
  - do not restrain the patient unless trained to do so;
  - never try to remove weapons from the patient.

Mental health disorders

- During the interview:
  - talk slowly, softly and clearly;
  - sympathize with the patient (without appearing patronizing);
  - maintain an attentive but relaxed posture;
  - allow the patient to talk, but do not let them talk themselves into an agitated state;
  - assess whether eye contact will appear threatening to patient or calming.
- Pharmacological therapy:
  - first line is oral drugs (as opposed to IM injections);
  - oral drugs:
    - lorazepam 1–2 mg ± haloperidol 5–10 mg,
    - have flumazenil to hand to reverse benzodiazepine-induced respiratory depression,
    - if using haloperidol always ensure that an antimuscarinic (e.g. procyclidine) is available in case of acute dystonia or other extrapyramidal side-effects (see the sections Neuroleptic malignant syndrome and Acute dystonic reaction above);
  - if oral drugs are refused or they are unsuccessful use intramuscular preparations:
    - lorazepam 1–2 mg (maximum 4–6 mg in 24 hours) ± haloperidol 5–10 mg (maximum 15 mg in 24 hours);
  - a second dose may then be necessary if this fails to control symptoms.

MICRO-facts

If it is anticipated that a patient is likely to become aggressive or agitated prescribe some lorazepam under the 'as needed' medication so that nursing staff can administer this in emergencies.

Mental health disorders

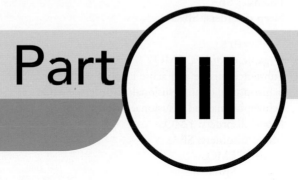

Part III

Self-assessment

16. Mental health assessment and service provision 237
  Questions 237
  History and examination: EMQs 237
  Mental health and the law: EMQs 238
  Multidisciplinary team: EMQs 239

  Answers 240
  History and examination: EMQs 240
  Mental health and the law: EMQs 241
  Multidisciplinary team: EMQs 242

17. Mental health disorders 243
  Questions 243
  Organic disorders: EMQs 243
  Substance misuse and acute alcohol withdrawal: SBAs 244
  Schizophrenia and delusional disorders: EMQs 244
  Schizophrenia and delusional disorders: SBAs 247
  Mood disorders: EMQs 248
  Mood disorders: SBAs 249
  Anxiety: EMQs 249
  Anxiety: SBAs 250
  Self-harm and suicide: EMQs 251
  Self-harm and suicide: SBA 251

Child and adolescent: SBA 252
Eating disorders: EMQs 252
Forensic: SBA 253
Sleep disorders: SBAs 253

Answers 254
Organic disorders: EMQs 254
Substance misuse and acute alcohol withdrawal: SBAs 254
Schizophrenia and delusional disorders: EMQs 255
Schizophrenia and delusional disorders: SBAs 256
Mood disorders: EMQs 257
Mood disorders: SBAs 257
Anxiety: EMQs 258
Anxiety: SBAs 258
Self-harm and suicide: EMQs 259
Self-harm and suicide: SBA 259
Child and adolescent: SBA 259
Eating disorders: EMQs 259
Forensic: SBA 260
Sleep disorders: SBAs 260

18. Treatment and psychiatric emergencies 261
Questions 261
Electroconvulsive therapy and psychotherapy: SBA 261
Lithium and mood stabilizers: SBAs 261
Antidepressants: EMQs 262
Antidepressants: SBA 262
Antipsychotics: EMQs 263
Acute dystonic reaction: SBA 263

Answers 264
Electroconvulsive therapy and psychotherapy: SBA 264
Lithium and mood stabilizers: SBAs 264
Antidepressants: EMQs 264
Antidepressants: SBA 265
Antipsychotics: EMQs 265
Acute dystonic reaction: SBA 265

Mental health assessment and service provision

Questions

HISTORY AND EXAMINATION: EMQs

For each of the following clinical scenarios please choose the most likely delusion type being expressed by the patient. Each option may be used once, more than once or not at all.

Delusion types

1) Grandiose
2) Hypochondriacal
3) Nihilistic
4) Of control (passivity phenomena)
5) Of guilt
6) Of jealousy
7) Of poverty
8) Of reference
9) Persecutory
10) Sexual delusion

Question 1

A 24-year-old female is brought to the emergency department (ED) by ambulance with a fractured left ankle having jumped from a high wall, claiming she had a number of special powers, including the ability to fly. She is wearing a bright, tight-fitting T-shirt and a net skirt. She loudly informs ED staff that she is a millionaire celebrity and a close relation of Mick Jagger.

Question 2

A 65-year-old man presents to his general practitioner (GP) convinced that his intestines are rotting away. He has a long-standing history of depression for which he has previously been treated with electroconvulsive therapy. On further questioning he reveals that everything around him is steadily disappearing into nothingness and he believes the world itself is going to come to an end very soon.

Question 3

You are a junior doctor working on a general surgical ward. One of your patients, a 77-year-old female who has undergone a bowel resection, calls you over to say that each time someone turns the light on or off in her room she knows that this is a coded message to her as she is an undercover spy. She asks you not to tell any of the other members of the team in case her cover is blown.

For each of the following clinical scenarios please choose the most likely diagnosis based on the clinical findings. Each option may be used once, more than once or not at all.

Diagnostic options

1) Acute cocaine intoxication
2) Anorexia nervosa
3) Binge-eating disorder
4) Borderline personality disorder
5) Lithium-induced hypothyroidism
6) Mixed anxiety and depressive disorder
7) Opiate overdose
8) Panic attack
9) Parkinsonism
10) Tricyclic overdose

Question 4

You are a junior doctor working a night shift in the ED and a 30-year-old male is brought into the department at 9 p.m. On examination you find that he has pin-point pupils, a Glasgow coma scale (GCS) of 8, bradycardia and respiratory depression. There are needle-track marks on his limbs. He also has numerous scars from previous superficial cutting on his left forearm and abdomen.

Question 5

You are a junior doctor working in general practice and a 35-year-old man comes to visit you complaining of tiredness and constipation. His voice is hoarse. Examination findings show that he is bradycardic, has put on weight and has a mild tremor.

Question 6

You are a junior doctor working in the Medical Assessment Unit and are asked to assess a 55-year-old female admitted with chest pain. On examination she is tachycardic and sweaty. She is shaky, feels nauseated and has tingling in both hands. Her blood pressure is 160/98 mmHg and her respiratory rate is increased. She tells you she feels short of breath and is terrified she is about to die.

MENTAL HEALTH AND THE LAW: EMQs

For each of the following clinical scenarios please choose the most appropriate option from the list below. Each alternative may be used once, more than once or not at all.

Options

1) Allow to self-discharge
2) Assess capacity
3) Assessment under the Mental Health Act (MHA)
4) Call police to detain patient
5) Community Treatment Order
6) Detain under Section 2
7) Detain under Section 3
8) Detain under Section 4
9) Detain under Section 5(2)
10) Do nothing

Question 7

You are a General Practice Vocational Training Scheme trainee working in the ED. A patient is brought in after being found in a stairwell with stab wounds. He tells you he did it to try and cut the evil out from inside him because otherwise the devil will not leave him alone. He is clearly responding to external stimuli. He wants to leave the ED and refuses to have anything to do with psychiatric services. He states that he will kill anyone who gets in his way when he tries to leave.

Question 8

You are called to the ward to see a 60-year-old man who wants to self-discharge. He was admitted 24 hours ago with pneumonia. He is shaking and says he can see little people in his room. In his notes you see he has a history of alcohol abuse.

Question 9

An elderly lady admitted after a bad fall says she wants to leave. The nurses say that she has been confused about where she is all day. They spoke to her neighbour earlier who said that she is normally fine and has no mental health problems.

MULTIDISCIPLINARY TEAM: EMQs

For each of the following descriptions/scenarios below choose from the list the correct service or team member best suited to deal with the clinical scenario. Each option may be used once, more than once or not at all.

Options

1) Assertive outreach team
2) Clinical psychologist
3) Crisis resolution and home treatment team
4) Early intervention
5) Occupational therapist
6) Pharmacist
7) Psychiatric nurse
8) Psychiatrist
9) Secretary
10) Social worker

Question 10

Which service is best suited to those patients that are in the community and have a new diagnosis of psychosis and require intensive support?

Question 11

Which team member is involved in the weekly ward rounds and provides key information on how the patient is managing on the ward on a day-to-day basis?

Question 12

You are a GP and a new patient is brought into your surgery by his mother. She is concerned as her son is showing increased concern that he is under surveillance by the police day and night. She has noticed that he seems distracted, withdrawn, and occasionally she has heard him talking to himself in an aggressive manner. You notice that he is unkempt, has poor eye contact and is stating that he hears a male voice telling him every day that he should kill himself.

You would like advice and support as you are gravely concerned for this patient's safety. He is not keen on going into hospital but is willing to accept psychiatric help.

Answers

HISTORY AND EXAMINATION: EMQs

Answer 1

1) **Grandiose.** This patient is likely to be having a manic episode. A number of features support this: bright and colourful clothing; loud, abnormal thought content. Patients with mania can express grandiose delusions. Here, these include beliefs about being able to fly and being a millionaire celebrity.

Answer 2

3) **Nihilistic.** This is the most likely delusional type that fits with both of his delusions, that his intestines are rotting and that the world is going to end. Nihilistic delusions occur in severe depression.

Answer 3

8) **Delusions of reference.** This patient is an elderly lady who is on a surgical ward post-bowel resection. She is demonstrating delusions of reference, as when one particular event occurs (the light switch) she relates that to a particular belief

(that she is an undercover spy). In her case it would be important to rule out delirium caused by, for example, infection or hypoxia.

Answer 4

7) **Opiate overdose.** Clues to let you know that this is likely to be an opiate overdose are the low GCS, pin-point pupils and the needle-track marks.

Answer 5

5) **Lithium-induced hypothyroidism.** Although there are no clues to state that this patient is taking lithium, except the tremor, the symptoms that he is presenting with are characteristic of hypothyroidism so it is therefore the most likely diagnosis from the list.

Answer 6

8) **Panic attack.** The examination findings seen in this case are indicative of a panic attack. Also, note the fact that she was admitted with chest pain, of which panic attack is a differential diagnosis. She is experiencing a heightened sense of anxiety and these clinical signs are typical.

MENTAL HEALTH AND THE LAW: EMQs

Answer 7

3) **Assessment under the MHA.** This patient is presenting as psychotic and is clearly a risk to himself and others. He needs to be assessed under the MHA. The most appropriate action is to request an assessment (as the patient is refusing to engage) with a view to detaining him for further assessment.

Answer 8

2) **Assess capacity.** The patient is either acutely confused from his infection and/or withdrawing from alcohol given his past history. Although he wants to self-discharge he should at the very least be assessed for capacity to make that decision and in all probability he will be found to lack capacity. The treating team can then treat him acting in his best interest. If he becomes acutely unwell then the treatment may be necessary to save his life.

Answer 9

2) **Assess capacity.** This lady appears to be suffering from delirium. Before she can be allowed to discharge herself her ability to make decisions must be checked.

MULTIDISCIPLINARY TEAM: EMQs

Answer 10

4) **Early intervention.** This patient has a new diagnosis of psychosis and is currently in the community. The early intervention service is for patients who require support in the first 2–3 years following a first episode of psychosis. It aims to promote early recovery from the illness.

Answer 11

7) **Psychiatric nurse.** Many of the members from the multidisciplinary team will be present at the weekly ward rounds, and a psychiatric nurse is best placed to describe how the patient is managing on the ward and whether there are any new concerns or areas that are improving.

Answer 12

3) **Crisis resolution and home treatment team.** This patient seems to have a new acute episode of psychosis. He currently has only presented to his general practitioner and has not been reviewed by a psychiatrist so a formal diagnosis is yet to be made. He is also a patient who may need to be admitted to an inpatient unit as he is expressing suicidal ideation. The crisis resolution and home treatment team would be a good place to start for advice as they will be able to formally assess the patient and determine whether he can be managed in the community or whether he needs to be admitted. The crisis resolution team usually includes a psychiatrist for medical input.

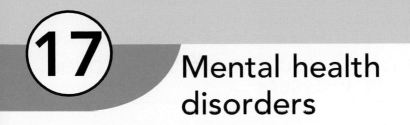

Mental health disorders

Questions

ORGANIC DISORDERS: EMQs

In the cases below choose the most likely diagnosis. Each option may be used once, more than once or not at all.

Diagnostic options

1) Dementia with human immunodeficiency virus (HIV) and acquired immune deficiency syndrome (AIDS)
2) Frontal lobe tumour
3) Hypercalcaemia
4) Korsakoff's syndrome
5) Multiple sclerosis
6) Temporal lobe abscess
7) Variant Creutzfeldt–Jakob disease
8) Viral encephalitis
9) Vitamin B12 deficiency
10) Wilson's disease

Question 1

A 55-year-old man is brought to see his general practitioner (GP) by his wife who reports he has become a completely different person over recent weeks. He recently lost his job for being rude to his customers and turning up late for work, which is completely out of character for the usually very pleasant and organized man. On examination he is incontinent of urine and has papilloedema.

Question 2

A 30-year-old woman comes to hospital after falling down the stairs. This is the second time this has happened in the last month. She says she has become quite unsteady while walking. She is otherwise well and her only previous attendance was to the emergency department (ED) when she lost the vision in her left eye for 3 days.

Question 3

A 45-year-old man is referred to hospital as he has become severely jaundiced. When the doctor tries to take a history the patient is frightened and agitated stating 'they are coming for me, they want to kill me this time'; he also accuses the nursing staff of plotting against him. You notice a ring around his cornea.

SUBSTANCE MISUSE AND ACUTE ALCOHOL WITHDRAWAL: SBAs

Question 4

If a man is said to be drinking harmfully how many units a week would he need to be drinking?
1) 25
2) 40
3) 50
4) 55
5) 60

Question 5

Which of the following is not part of the management of a patient who is acutely withdrawing from alcohol?
1) A reducing regime of chlordiazepoxide
2) Acamprosate
3) Multivitamins
4) Regular monitoring of vital signs
5) Thiamine/Pabrinex

SCHIZOPHRENIA AND DELUSIONAL DISORDERS: EMQs

For each of the following clinical scenarios please choose the most likely diagnosis. Each option may be used once, more than once or not at all.

Diagnostic options

1) Acute polymorphic disorder without symptoms of schizophrenia
2) Acute schizophrenia-like disorder
3) Alcohol abuse disorder
4) De Clérambault's syndrome
5) Hyperthyroidism
6) Induced delusional disorder
7) Paranoid schizophrenia
8) Persecutory delusional disorder
9) Residual schizophrenia
10) Schizoaffective disorder: manic type

Question 6

You are a junior doctor in psychiatry. In clinic you see a 29-year-old woman who is referred to you urgently by her GP with a 10-day history of sudden-onset persistent persecutory delusions and second-person auditory hallucinations which are interfering with her ability to function on a day-to-day basis. She tells you that she has had a tough few weeks as her father has recently died.

Question 7

You are a junior doctor on the psychiatric ward. A 33-year-old woman is referred to you with a 3-month history of progressive paranoid symptoms coupled with excess energy and elation. On assessment she tells you that she has lost 2 stone (12.7 kg) since the beginning of the symptoms. On examination you notice that she has an irregularly irregular pulse.

Question 8

You are a junior doctor in psychiatry. A 45-year-old man is referred to your clinic by his GP. When he arrives it is clear that he is not happy to be here. He tells you that his next door neighbour (who is a keen birdwatcher) is 'out to get him'. He says that this all started 6 months ago after he saw him looking at him 'in a funny way'. Your patient says that he is convinced that he is going to be murdered in his sleep and a confrontation 2 months ago ended in violence. He is making arrangements to sue his neighbour for breach of privacy.

For each of the following clinical scenarios please choose the most useful investigation to aid diagnosis. Although all of these tests should be used in investigation of a psychotic patient please choose the answer that is most likely to yield a positive result. Each option may be used once, more than once or not at all.

Options

1) Computed tomography (CT)
2) Electrocardiogram (ECG)
3) Electroencephalogram (EEG)
4) Full blood count (FBC)
5) Liver function tests (LFTs)
6) Serum calcium and parathyroid hormone (PTH)
7) Syphilis screen
8) Urea and electrolytes (U&E)
9) Urine drug screen
10) Vitamin B_1

Question 9

A 63-year-old woman on a medical ward with a catheter in place suddenly develops visual hallucinations accompanied by excess drowsiness. The staff on her ward report that she has been verbally aggressive to anyone who approaches her and that her speech is incoherent.

Question 10

A 24-year-old unemployed man who spends most of his time partying develops persistent auditory hallucinations and delusions of reference. He tells you that he had an unhappy childhood, never got on with his parents and left school aged 16 years. He has a past history of amphetamine use.

Question 11

A 42-year-old male is admitted onto the psychiatry ward. He is well known to the services having suffered from schizophrenia for 20 years, and despite being on depot antipsychotic medication he says that he is still hearing voices and getting very anxious about the fact that the Government is trying to have him assassinated because he has top secret plans to dig a tunnel from his back garden to China. He has a long history of heavy alcohol use, and currently drinks 3 L of cider a day. He had a recent blood test for suspected anaemia but the full blood count was entirely normal.

In the cases below choose the investigation that would most likely help you diagnose a cause for a patient's delirium. Each option may be used once, more than once or not at all.

Options

1) Blood glucose
2) C-Reactive protein
3) HIV test
4) LFTs
5) Lumbar puncture
6) Mid-stream urine
7) Urinary Na^+
8) Pelvic X-ray
9) Serum B_{12} and folate
10) U&E

Question 12

A 75-year-old woman is found by her daughter semi-conscious lying on the floor. She is incoherent and is unable to say what has happened. This has happened on a few occasions before. She has been unwell for a few days and has not been eating, although she was still managing to drink lots of water.

Question 13

A 68-year-old man is on your ward 1 day after a knee replacement. He was previously well but since his operation has been confused, disorientated and aggressive to staff. His blood pressure, temperature and SaO_2 (oxygen saturation) are normal. He is on regular non-steroidal anti-inflammatory drugs (NSAIDs) for post-operative pain relief as well as medication for hypertension, high cholesterol and type 2 diabetes.

Question 14

A 52-year-old man is admitted to a medical ward after being brought in by ambulance. He says that he was having a drink earlier that morning at the Working Men's Club when he started to have chest pain. Two days following his admission psychiatry input is requested as the patient has started to report that he can see people in his room, although there is no-one there. When seen, he is agitated, confused, shaky and complaining of nausea. He is not on any regular medication, had been declared medically fit and was due to be discharged. He lost his job 6 months ago and tells you this was because he kept missing work.

SCHIZOPHRENIA AND DELUSIONAL DISORDERS: SBAs

Question 15

Which of the following is not one of Schneider's first-rank symptoms?
1) Delusional perception
2) Made feelings
3) Thought echo
4) Thought insertion
5) Visual hallucinations

Question 16

You are the psychiatry doctor on call. You receive a referral from the ED, with very little information apart from the fact that the patient is a 32-year-old agitated and aggressive female showing 'clinical features consistent with schizophrenia'. Before the patient comes up you formulate a list of potential differential diagnoses from the little information that you have been given. Which of the following is not going to be on your list?
1) Catatonic schizophrenia
2) Hebephrenic schizophrenia
3) Paranoid schizophrenia
4) Residual schizophrenia
5) Simple schizophrenia

Question 17

Which of the following statements about delirium is false?
1) Consciousness is impaired
2) Insomnia is a common feature
3) Sleep–wake cycle is disturbed
4) Symptoms are typically worse first thing in the morning
5) Tactile hallucinations can occur

Question 18

A 20-year-old woman presents suffering with palpitations and episodic severe anxiety. She has been sweating a lot recently and feels that her heart is always racing. When you take her pulse it is 115 beats/minute. She reports that she started taking ramipril and amlodipine daily 3 weeks ago. Which of the tests below is likely to give a cause for this lady's symptoms?

1) Adrenocorticotropic hormone (ACTH) stimulation test
2) Measure urinary catecholamines
3) Thyroid-stimulating hormone (TSH)
4) Triiodothyronine (T_3)/thyroxine (T_4)
5) 24-hour urinary cortisol test

MOOD DISORDERS: EMQs

For each of the following clinical scenarios please choose the most likely diagnosis. Each option may be used once, more than once or not at all.

Diagnostic options

1) Bipolar affective disorder, current episode hypomanic
2) Bipolar affective disorder, current episode mild depression with somatic syndrome
3) Bipolar affective disorder, current episode moderate depression without somatic syndrome
4) Bipolar affective disorder, current episode severe depression with psychotic symptoms
5) Bipolar affective disorder, current episode manic with psychotic symptoms
6) Cyclothymia
7) Dysthymia
8) Hypomanic episode
9) Mild depressive episode with somatic syndrome
10) Recurrent depression, currently in remission

Question 19

A 19-year-old woman comes to see you with a 2-week history of low mood, anhedonia, recurrent nocturnal awakenings, feelings of guilt and suicidal ideation. She tells you that a year ago she had a 3-week period of intense euphoria, increased energy, grandiosity and poor concentration.

Question 20

A 23-year-old man comes to see you after yelling at his boss at work. He says that for the past 3 days he has not needed to sleep much, he feels full of energy but has been feeling 'up and down' in his mood.

Question 21

A 22-year-old woman comes to you with a 2-year history of chronically low mood, fatigue and low self-esteem, but without suicidal ideation. She says she has 'some good days' but these do not last very long.

MOOD DISORDERS: SBAs

Question 22

Which of the following signs would you definitely **not** expect to see on mental state examination of a patient presenting with a moderate depressive episode?
1) Delusions of persecution
2) Monotonous voice
3) Psychomotor agitation
4) Tangentiality
5) Weight loss

Question 23

Which of the following drugs is appropriate as the first drug therapy for a patient presenting with their first episode of moderate depression with somatic syndrome?
1) Amitriptyline
2) Aripiprazole
3) Fluoxetine
4) Lithium
5) Mirtazapine

ANXIETY: EMQs

For each of the following clinical scenarios please choose the most appropriate diagnosis from the list below. Each option may be used once, more than once or not at all.

Options

1) Acute stress disorder
2) Adjustment disorder
3) Agoraphobia
4) Generalized anxiety disorder (GAD)
5) Hyperthyroidism
6) Mixed anxiety and depression
7) Obsessive–compulsive disorder (OCD)
8) Panic disorder
9) Post-traumatic stress disorder (PTSD)
10) Social phobia

Question 24

A 27-year-old ex-soldier is brought into the ED after being found unconscious outside a pub smelling of alcohol. He is sleeping in a bay when there is a large bang as a door slams. He wakes up and jumps under his bed to shelter. He then falls back asleep but keeps shouting 'Don't shoot me, don't shoot'. His parents who have accompanied him, tell you he has not been himself since coming back from his last tour of duty in Afghanistan where several of his friends were killed.

Question 25

A 45-year-old man visits his GP. He has recently been promoted at work and is now involved in training new employees. He is worried that his new job is too stressful as every time he has run a training session he gets palpitations and feels nauseated and dizzy.

Question 26

A patient you have seen many times before comes to see you as she is having trouble sleeping. She feels uneasy all the time but says nothing has changed in her life recently. At night she is worrying about her son, work and finances but on further questioning there is nothing in particular on her mind.

ANXIETY: SBAs

Question 27

A previously well 25-year-old woman presents with episodes of chest pain and dizziness. It can come on at any time and she is worried it is serious as it feels as if she is going to die. You think she may be suffering from panic disorder. What is the most appropriate investigation?
1) An echocardiogram (ECG)
2) Blood glucose
3) Cholesterol level
4) Nothing
5) Thyroid function tests (TFTs)

Question 28

A patient has become obsessed with the idea of death and is very distressed by this. He tells you he has to turn the light switch on and off 20 times before he can leave a room so that no-one dies. Which of the features below would not support a diagnosis of OCD?
1) He believes someone is putting these thoughts inside his head
2) He gets upset when thinking about carrying out the rituals
3) He is still going to work each day
4) The actions have been successfully hidden from his family
5) The patient tries unsuccessfully to resist performing the ritual

SELF-HARM AND SUICIDE: EMQs

For each of the following questions please choose the most appropriate answer from the options below. Each alternative may be used once, more than once or not at all.

Options

1) ABCDE assessment
2) Cognitive behavioural therapy (CBT)
3) Counselling
4) Detain under Mental Health Act
5) Discharge
6) Medical admission
7) Psychiatric assessment
8) Surgical assessment
9) Toxicology screen (paracetamol, etc.)
10) Treat for depression

Question 29

A 50-year-old man is brought in by ambulance to the ED. He is bleeding profusely from two large cuts, one on each wrist. He is conscious and tells you he cut his wrists deliberately and wanted to die. As you are talking to him he becomes dizzy and loses consciousness. Which action should be taken first?

Question 30

A 16-year-old girl is brought in by her mother who found her lying on the bathroom floor. She is covered in vomit and her mother says there was an empty bottle of vodka next to her. She is confused and not answering questions. What action would you take first?

Question 31

You see a 30-year-old woman and her friend in the ED. She has a cut down one wrist which has already been sutured. Her friend tells you that the patient has been very depressed since her sister was killed in a car accident 2 months ago. When you ask the patient she says it was a silly mistake and she only did it because she was drunk and felt sad. She wants to go home. What is the most appropriate action to take?

SELF-HARM AND SUICIDE: SBA

Question 32

A 50-year-old man is brought into the ED. He was found in his bath with his wrists cut by his cleaner who came 3 hours earlier than usual. He is not answering questions but the cleaner gives you a note she found and tells you his wife recently left him and he is unemployed. She also tells you she has found many empty vodka bottles in the rubbish and knows he has been low in mood lately. Your Registrar asks you to score the patient and work out which category of risk he is in. Choose the single best answer to the scenario:

1) High risk − 9
2) Low risk − 2
3) Medium risk − 7
4) Unable to assess

CHILD AND ADOLESCENT: SBA

Question 33

Which of the following statements about attention-deficit hyperactivity disorder is false?

1) A common symptom is the inability to listen
2) Features get worse as the child enters adolescence
3) It is commonly associated with conduct disorder
4) Symptoms must be present before the age of 6 years
5) The condition is commonly treated with psychostimulant medication

EATING DISORDERS: EMQs

For each of the clinical scenarios described below, choose the most likely diagnosis. Each option may be used once, more than once or not at all.

Options

1) Addison's disease
2) Anorexia nervosa
3) Bipolar disorder
4) Borderline personality disorder
5) Bulimia nervosa
6) Coeliac disease
7) Depression
8) Hypoglycaemia
9) OCD
10) Pregnancy

Question 34

A 17-year-old female presented to her GP as she was worried about her recent weight loss. She stated that she had lost nearly 3 stones (19 kg) in 6 months and her current body mass index (BMI) was only 16. When questioned she denied trying to lose weight herself. She did however admit to 'abnormal' eating habits, finding she could only eat food at set times of the day and all food items always had to be laid out in exactly the same way on her plate. When asked why this was the case she stated that bad things would happen if she didn't stick to these rules.

Question 35

A 14-year-old female was brought to her GP as her mother was concerned about her weight. She had dropped around 2 stone (12.7 kg) in only 2 months, although she was not worried about it. Her current BMI was 17. When asked about her eating habits she did not volunteer much information but her mother stated she hardly ate anything, pushed food around the plate and she would find food in her room under the bed. On examination she was cold and pale. She had fine hair over her body and she was no longer menstruating.

Question 36

A 20-year-old female came to her general practitioner as she had noticed that her weight had dropped recently by about half a stone (3.2 kg). She was also finding that she was suffering with diarrhoea on occasion. She was feeling increasingly tired. On examination she looked pale and had cool peripheries. She also reported feeling bloated. Her calculated BMI was 18.

FORENSIC: SBA

Question 37

Which of the following is true for a diminished responsibility plea?
1) Is only valid if the patient has schizophrenia
2) Can reduce an offence of murder to manslaughter
3) Means that a custodial sentence is avoided
4) The patient must have a reduced IQ
5) The sentence, if any, can only be carried out in a secure psychiatric unit

SLEEP DISORDERS: SBAs

Question 38

A 60-year-old woman presents with problems sleeping. She has not slept well for years but feels that it has got much worse over the last month. She wants you to give her something to make her sleep. What is the most appropriate action?
1) Advise about sleep hygiene
2) Prescribe benzodiazepines
3) Prescribe zopiclone
4) Refer for CBT
5) Refer to sleep centre

Question 39

Which of the following is not a cause of insomnia?
1) Depression
2) Exercise
3) Gastric reflux
4) Heart failure
5) Snoring

Answers

ORGANIC DISORDERS: EMQs

Answer 1

2) **Frontal lobe tumour.** A change in behaviour with loss of ability to plan. Labile mood and inability to control actions all point towards frontal lobe pathology.

Answer 2

5) **Multiple sclerosis.** A young woman with neurological symptoms such as ataxia and clumsiness. A previous episode of optic neuritis was described. Two episodes mean that she meets the clinical criteria for multiple sclerosis.

Answer 3

10) **Wilson's disease.** Jaundice with symptoms of psychosis demonstrates both hepatic and central nervous system involvement. The Kayser–Fleischer ring around the cornea is a classical sign in Wilson's disease, which affects both systems.

SUBSTANCE MISUSE AND ACUTE ALCOHOL WITHDRAWAL: SBAs

Answer 4

3) **50 units.** For a man to be said to be drinking harmfully he needs to be drinking at least 50 units of alcohol weekly. For women it is 35 units or more weekly.

Answer 5

2) **Acamprosate.** This is a drug that is used in the long-term management of a patient who is dependent on alcohol. It is not indicated in the management of acute withdrawal from alcohol. It is used to suppress the cravings of alcohol.

SCHIZOPHRENIA AND DELUSIONAL DISORDERS: EMQs

Answer 6

2) **Acute schizophrenia-like disorder.** This patient has been suffering from delusions and auditory hallucinations, which are all symptoms of schizophrenia; however, the sudden onset suggests a diagnosis of an acute and transient psychotic disorder. This will remain the preferred diagnosis unless the patient's symptoms last longer than 1 month. The acute onset following a psychosocial stressor (her father's death) also points to this diagnosis.

Answer 7

5) **Hyperthyroidism.** The presence of both schizophrenic and manic symptoms could suggest a diagnosis of schizoaffective disorder: manic type. However, the weight loss and irregularly irregular pulse (atrial fibrillation) point to hyperthyroidism, particularly given the patient's sex and age. At the very least, this would be the most important condition to rule out as the cause of her psychosis.

Answer 8

8) **Persecutory delusional disorder.** This man is suffering from paranoid delusions and, given his age and lack of other symptoms, a delusional disorder would be the appropriate diagnosis. The fact that he is about to engage in formal legal action over his symptoms is characteristic of this disorder.

Answer 9

4) **FBC.** This woman is suffering from delirium, most likely secondary to an ascending urinary tract infection from her catheter. The visual hallucinations, impaired consciousness, aggression, disorientation and incoherence are all characteristic of delirium. A FBC would confirm the presence of infection.

Answer 10

9) **Urine drug screen.** The cause of this man's psychosis is most likely illicit drug use. By obtaining a urine test the drug of abuse can be confirmed.

Self-assessment

Answer 11

5) **LFTs.** This man already has a diagnosis of schizophrenia; however, as he is still having symptoms a switch to clozapine (used very successfully for treatment resistant schizophrenia) should be considered. Before starting this drug LFTs need to be performed as clozapine can cause major liver problems. This is especially important for this man because of his history of heavy alcohol use. A FBC would also be important, as the drug can cause agranulocytosis.

Answer 12

1) **Blood glucose.** It is likely this patient is hypoglycaemic as she has not been eating. Any patient that is in a delirious state should have their blood glucose checked before any other investigation is performed to rule out hypoglycaemia or hyperglycaemia.

Answer 13

10) **U&E.** The patient has been started on regular NSAIDs, which are nephrotoxic, as well as his normal medication. This could lead to acute kidney injury. It is important that his renal function is checked and his medications are reviewed.

Answer 14

9) **Serum B_{12} and folate.** This man was admitted from a Working Men's Club in the morning and lost his job 6 months ago. It is likely he has been drinking heavily during this period given the history and he is now in withdrawal following his admission. This is the most likely reason for his hallucinations and delirium. He could also be folate-, thiamine- and B_{12}-deficient and it is important that this is picked up early and appropriate treatment is given to avoid the development of long-term complications.

SCHIZOPHRENIA AND DELUSIONAL DISORDERS: SBAs

Answer 15

5) **Visual hallucinations.** Although auditory hallucinations are included in Schneider's first-rank symptoms, visual hallucinations are not. All of the other options are included.

Answer 16

2) **Hebephrenic schizophrenia.** Although you do not have any information that can help you pin down the correct diagnosis, the age of the patient

automatically rules out a diagnosis of hebephrenic schizophrenia, as this subtype is only seen in the adolescent to young adult age group.

Answer 17

4) **Symptoms are typically worse first thing in the morning.** This is false; delirium symptoms are usually worse in the evening and at night.

Answer 18

2) **Measure urinary catecholamines.** This is a young woman presenting with tachycardia, palpitations and sweating. The medications she is on indicate she has hypertension which is unusual at her age. The high blood pressure with these symptoms points to a phaeochromocytoma rather that hyperthyroidism which would not cause the hypertension.

MOOD DISORDERS: EMQs

Answer 19

3) **Bipolar affective disorder, current episode moderate depression without somatic syndrome.** Given the depressed nature of the current episode and the manic features of the previous episode, bipolar affective disorder is the correct diagnosis. This woman has two of the core symptoms of depression plus three of the secondary symptoms with only one of somatic syndrome, which gives this episode a diagnosis of moderate depression without somatic syndrome.

Answer 20

8) **Hypomanic episode.** This man has only a 3-day history of manic symptoms. He is still able to go into work, which suggests that the disturbance to everyday life is not complete. He may go on to have a manic episode within bipolar disorder, but hypomanic episode is the correct diagnosis at this point.

Answer 21

7) **Dysthymia.** This lady has a chronically low mood with other depressive symptoms; however, these are not sufficient to diagnose a depressive disorder. Dysthymia is the correct diagnosis in this case.

MOOD DISORDERS: SBAs

Answer 22

4) **Tangentiality.** This is a manifestation of flight of ideas, a form of thought disorder that is not usually seen in moderate depression. The other symptoms may be apparent in a patient with moderate depression.

Answer 23

3) **Fluoxetine.** Fluoxetine is a selective serotonin re-uptake inhibitor (SSRI) which is the first-line therapy for patients with depression. The other drugs are useful for second-line therapy or as adjuvant therapy.

ANXIETY: EMQs

Answer 24

9) **PTSD.** The patient has a history of exposure to traumatic events, is sensitive to loud noises and is possibly having nightmares. These are all symptoms of PTSD. It appears the patient is abusing alcohol, which is a common way of coping with this disorder.

Answer 25

10) **Social phobia.** The patient is having symptoms of a panic attack which occur when talking in front of others. This is a presentation of social phobia that is common in men and may not present until the patient is put in a situation that involves public speaking.

Answer 26

4) **GAD.** The patient has a free-floating anxiety that is leaving her unable to fall asleep. Although she is worried about many things there is no particular worry, which points to a generalized anxiety rather than a specific phobia.

ANXIETY: SBAs

Answer 27

5) **TFTs.** Although the episodes sound like panic attacks they could also be a new presentation of hyperthyroidism. It is important to check thyroid function and order an ECG to rule out organic causes so you can reassure the patient and treat the panic disorders.

Answer 28

1) **He believes someone is putting these thoughts inside his head.** In order to be diagnosed with OCD a patient must know they are carrying out the actions themselves and not believe they are the result of an outside force. All of the other answers support a diagnosis of OCD.

SELF-HARM AND SUICIDE: EMQs

Answer 29

1) ABCDE assessment. This patient is actively bleeding on arrival and has now lost consciousness. He is therefore haemodynamically unstable and needs to be assessed using the ABC framework. Once he has been appropriately resuscitated and is stable a psychiatric assessment would be important.

Answer 30

9) Toxicology screen. Although this girl has consumed a large amount of alcohol, as she is unresponsive it is impossible to know what else she has taken so the first action should be to request a toxicology screen for paracetamol, salicylate levels and other drugs to determine if she needs treatment for an overdose.

Answer 31

7) Psychiatric assessment. Although this patient is medically ready for discharge, all patients who attempt suicide/self-harm need a psychiatric assessment before leaving the ED.

SELF-HARM AND SUICIDE: SBA

Answer 32

1) High risk—9. This patient is at high risk of another attempt as he had left a suicide note and was found by chance. He is a separated, unemployed, middle-aged man. All of these put him into the high-risk category.

CHILD AND ADOLESCENT: SBA

Answer 33

2) Features get worse as the child enters adolescence. The opposite is actually true, symptoms normally improve as the child gets older; however, in severe cases symptoms may persist into adolescence.

EATING DISORDERS: EMQs

Answer 34

9) OCD. This patient has a low BMI at only 16 which would fit with anorexia. However, the history that she gives fits more with OCD; unfortunately, her compulsive acts are related to food. Treatment of her OCD should see an increase in her weight. An SSRI would be appropriate.

Answer 35

2) **Anorexia nervosa.** This history is typical of anorexia nervosa. The young female does not feel that her weight is of any concern but other family members are concerned and have noticed a dramatic drop in her weight. A BMI of 17 also fits the criteria for anorexia nervosa. Examination findings are also consistent with anorexia nervosa: the lanugo hair and the clinical signs of anaemia. Amenorrhoea is also a typical feature of anorexia nervosa in women because of a low level of oestrogen as fat stores are reduced.

Answer 36

6) **Coeliac disease.** This patient has typical symptoms of coeliac disease. The weight loss results from the malabsorption caused by the coeliac disease. Examination findings are consistent with anaemia which is caused by malabsorption of iron, leading to iron-deficiency anaemia. A gluten-free diet would allow the small bowel to recover and the weight loss should resolve.

FORENSIC: SBA

Answer 37

2) **Can reduce an offence of murder to manslaughter.** A diminished responsibility plea is a murder defence which, if accepted, can reduce the offence to manslaughter. There are many cases where psychiatric conditions other than paranoid schizophrenia have been held to amount to diminished responsibility. These include depression, morbid jealousy and paranoid personality disorder.

SLEEP DISORDERS: SBAs

Answer 38

1) **Advise about sleep hygiene.** This patient is presenting with chronic insomnia. The first course of action is to give advice about sleep hygiene and then other options such as CBT could be considered. Medication should not be given for chronic insomnia and sleep centres should only be used if there is thought to be a physical cause.

Answer 39

2) **Exercise.** All of the others could cause insomnia whereas regular exercise during the day should improve a patient's sleep pattern.

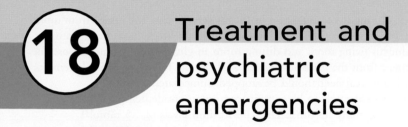

Treatment and psychiatric emergencies

Questions

ELECTROCONVULSIVE THERAPY AND PSYCHOTHERAPY: SBA

Question 1

Which of the following conditions are an indication for electroconvulsive therapy (ECT)?
1) Catatonic state
2) Dementia
3) Mild depressive illness
4) Obsessive-compulsive disorder (OCD)
5) Psychosis

LITHIUM AND MOOD STABILIZERS: SBAs

Question 2

Which of the following is not a typical feature of lithium toxicity?
1) Ataxia
2) Coarse tremor
3) Palpitations
4) Seizures
5) Vomiting

Question 3

You are a junior doctor in psychiatry and are assisting in your consultant's outpatient clinic. You see a 40-year-old man with a diagnosis of bipolar affective disorder who was started on lithium 9 months previously and had been on a stable dose. You notice that he is wearing shorts and flip-flops in the middle of winter. During the consultation he speaks very quickly and jumps from topic to topic. He states that he is looking forward to the weekend as he is planning to re-paint his living room and dining room in glittery-gold paint. Choose the statement from the list below which best fits the following clinical scenario:

1) Lithium treatment should be stopped immediately
2) The patient needs to be commenced on an antidepressant medication
3) The symptoms are consistent with lithium levels of 1.5 mmol/L
4) The symptoms are consistent with lithium levels of 0.2 mmol/L
5) The symptoms are likely caused by a psychotic episode

ANTIDEPRESSANTS: EMQs

For each of the following questions please choose the most appropriate drug. Each option may be used once, more than once or not at all.

Options

1) Amitriptyline
2) Citalopram
3) Fluoxetine
4) Isocarboxazid
5) Mirtazapine

6) Moclobemide
7) Phenelzine
8) Sertraline
9) Tranylcypromine
10) Venlafaxine

Question 4

This drug is licensed for use in bulimia nervosa and exerts its main action by blocking the re-uptake of serotonin at the level of the presynaptic membrane.

Question 5

This drug blocks the re-uptake of various neurotransmitters without much effect on histaminergic H_1 receptors.

Question 6

This drug is **not** suitable for a 50-year-old depressed bus driver who is a known sufferer of hepatitis C.

ANTIDEPRESSANTS: SBA

Question 7

Which of the following is not an anticholinergic side-effect of tricyclic antidepressants (TCAs)?

1) Blurred vision
2) Constipation
3) Dry mouth
4) Urinary retention
5) Vomiting

ANTIPSYCHOTICS: EMQs

For each of the following questions please choose the most appropriate side-effect of the antipsychotics being described. Each option may be used once, more than once or not at all.

Options

1) Acute dystonic reaction
2) Agranulocytosis
3) Akathisia
4) Amenorrhoea
5) Galactorrhoea
6) Neuroleptic malignant syndrome
7) Osteoporosis
8) Photosensitivity
9) Postural hypotension
10) Tardive dyskinesia

Question 8

A patient on long-term antipsychotic treatment develops odd movements of their mouth, including lip smacking, puckering and tongue protrusion.

Question 9

A patient taking clozapine describes feeling dizzy on standing.

Question 10

A patient taking chlorpromazine develops a rash after spending a weekend at the beach.

ACUTE DYSTONIC REACTION: SBA

Question 11

A patient presents with a 1-week history of 'neck twisting' and is very distressed. You find out he was started on a new medication for his schizophrenia a few days ago. What is the most appropriate action?
1) Admit patient
2) Give IM procyclidine
3) Give propranolol
4) Reassure the patient only
5) Stop the medication

Answers

ELECTROCONVULSIVE THERAPY AND PSYCHOTHERAPY: SBA

Answer 1

1) **Catatonic state.** Catatonia not responding to benzodiazepines is an indication for ECT. Other indications would be severe mania or depression not responding to pharmacotherapy.

LITHIUM AND MOOD STABILIZERS: SBAs

Answer 2

3) **Palpitations.** Palpitations are not a typical feature of lithium toxicity. All the other features on the list are.

Answer 3

4) **The symptoms are consistent with lithium levels of 0.2 mmol/L.** The patient is displaying features of a manic episode. As the patient was previously stable, his relapse may result from non-compliance with medications at the prescribed dose. Patients often reduce or stop taking psychotropics when they have been well for a while and this leads to relapses. Here the patient is likely to be taking a sub-therapeutic dose hence the low serum lithium level.

ANTIDEPRESSANTS: EMQs

Answer 4

3) **Fluoxetine.** This drug is a selective serotonin re-uptake inhibitor that is licensed for use in bulimia nervosa as well as depression.

Answer 5

10) **Venlafaxine.** This drug is a selective serotonin and noradrenaline re-uptake inhibitor that has little effect on histaminergic H_1 receptors.

Answer 6

1) **Amitriptyline.** This drug is a TCA which means that it is contraindicated in severe liver disease, such as hepatitis C. It also has widely recognized sedative

effects, which would make this drug unsuitable for a patient whose main occupation is driving.

ANTIDEPRESSANTS: SBA

Answer 7

5) **Vomiting.** Although vomiting is a side-effect of TCAs, it is not attributable to its anticholinergic effect.

ANTIPSYCHOTICS: EMQs

Answer 8

10) **Tardive dyskinesia.** This is a typical presentation of rhythmic movements involving the facial muscles occurring after long-term use of usually typical antipsychotics.

Answer 9

9) **Postural hypotension.** Although clozapine is more commonly associated with the side-effects of agranulocytosis and hypersalivation, postural hypotension is among its listed side-effects.

Answer 10

8) **Photosensitivity.** Chlorpromazine typically causes a blue/grey photosensitive rash to occur.

ACUTE DYSTONIC REACTION: SBA

Answer 11

2) **Give IM procyclidine.** The patient is suffering from an acute dystonic reaction. He should be given IM procyclidine and it should be prescribed daily. His antipsychotics need to be reviewed.

Index

Note: 'vs' indicates the distinction or differential diagnosis of conditions. Page numbers with brackets e.g. 286(288–9), are to questions with the answer indicated in brackets. On some occasions with EMQs, the indexed topic does not appear in the question itself but is listed in the options on a preceding page.

ABCDE approach 251(259)
  acute substance intoxication 65
  overdose 220
abdominal examination 17
abuse (from others), risk of 16
acamprosate 68, 244(255)
acetylcholinesterase inhibitors,
    Alzheimer's disease 45
acute and transient psychotic disorders
    93–6, 245(255)
acute dystonic reaction 227–8,
    263(265)
acute episodes (and their management)
    mania 103–4
    schizophrenia 87
acute stress reaction 134–5
acute withdrawal state, alcohol 67,
    228–31, 244(255)
Addison's disease 57
adjustment disorder 137
administrator 25
adolescents 185–8, 252(259)
    depression 185–6, 193
    self-harm and suicide 186–7
    substance misuse 187–8
adoption studies
    bipolar affective disorder 116
    depressive episode 105
    schizophrenia 79
adrenergic pathways
    antidepressant effects 195
    panic disorder and 126

affect, assessment 11
affective (mood) disorders 100–22,
    248–9(257–8)
    criminal offences and 190
    substance abuse-related 71, 103
    see also schizoaffective disorders
age, dementia and 39
    Alzheimer's disease 42
    vascular dementia 45
aggression 231–3
agitation 231–3
    haloperidol in 38, 231, 233
    in neuroleptic malignant
        syndrome 226
    pharmacotherapy 38, 231, 233
agoraphobia 129–30
AIDS see HIV and AIDS-associated
    disorders
alcohol (overconsumption) 228–31,
    244(254–5), 247(256)
    acute intoxication 64–6
    acute withdrawal state 67, 228–31,
        244(255)
    criminal offences and 190–1
    dependency 62–3, 67–8, 70, 231
    detoxification 68, 230–1
    fetal consequences 175
    history-taking 8, 62–3
aliphatic side-chain phenothiazines 200,
    203
allergies, history-taking 5
Alzheimer's disease 42–5

Alzheimer's disease(*contd*)
  frontotemporal dementia vs 49
  risperidone in 41
amitriptyline 262(264–5)
amnesia
  in electroconvulsive therapy 214
  in head injury 55
amnesic syndrome (Wernicke–Korsakoff
    syndrome) 60, 71–3
amyloid precursor protein gene and
    Alzheimer's disease 43
anankastic personality disorder 132,
    163, 167
anergia 107
anhedonia 107
anorexia nervosa 142–5, 253(260)
anticholinergic effects
  antidepressants 195, 262–3(265)
  antipsychotics 203
anticholinesterases, Alzheimer's
    disease 45
antidepressants 193–7, 262–3(264–5)
  agoraphobia 130
  bipolar affective disorder 118
  bulimia nervosa 146
  depressive episode 105, 112, 249(258)
    adolescents 186, 193
    late-onset 51–2
    postnatal 158
  dysthymia 120
  generalised anxiety disorder 125, 212
  mechanisms of action 192, 194, 195,
    196, 198
  obsessive–compulsive disorder 134
  panic disorder 128, 212
  personality disorders 169
  postnatal psychosis 159
  post-traumatic stress syndrome 136
  in pregnancy 160
  social phobia 131
  starting/switching/stopping 193–4
antiepileptics as mood stabilizers 206,
    207
antioxidants and Alzheimer's disease 43
antipsychotics 197–205, 263(265)
  acute and transient psychotic
    disorders 95

postnatal psychosis 159
  atypical 203–4
  delusional disorders 92
    induced 97
  dementia 41
  depot 205
  depression 112
  general information 197–9
  manic episode 103
  newer 204–5
  personality disorders 169
  in pregnancy 160
  schizophrenia 80, 87
    late-onset 50
  side-effects 199, 201–3, 204, 205,
    263(265)
    extrapyramidal 38, 50, 87, 95, 160,
      201, 233
    neuroleptic malignant syndrome
      201, 202, 225–7
  starting/switching/stopping 199
  typical 200–3
antisocial personality disorder 163,
    165
anxiety and neuroses 123–41,
    249–50(258)
  learning disability and screening
    for 173
anxiolytics 209–12
  generalised anxiety disorder 125
anxious (cluster C) personality disorders
    163, 167, 168, 169
apathy, schizophrenia 85
apolipoprotein E gene and Alzheimer's
    disease 43
appearance, assessment 9, 15
aripiprazole 97, 204
ascorbate (vitamin C) and Alzheimer's
    disease 43
Asperger's syndrome 182–3
assertive outreach teams 27
assessment (psychiatric/mental health)
    3–20, 237–8(240–1), 251(259)
  admission for 22
  in emergency 22
  children 176
  forensic patient 189

attachment (childhood)
  disorder 178–9
  normal 179
attention, assessment 14
attention deficit–hyperactivity
    (hyperkinetic) disorder 16, 179–80,
    252(259)
auditory hallucinations 11
  schizophrenia 83, 84
autism 180–2
autoimmune disorders 60–1
autonomic dysfunction, somatoform 140
autonomic symptoms
  in alcohol withdrawal 229
  in generalised anxiety disorder 124
  in neuroleptic malignant
      syndrome 226
avoidant personality disorder 163, 167

baby blues 155–6
bedwetting 184–5
behaviour
  abnormalities
    children 176–80
    dementia 40
    mania 101
  assessment 9, 15
  your, agitated/aggressive patients and
      paying attention to 232
behavioural syndromes associated with
    physiological disorders 142–61
behavioural therapy
  depression, for couples 112
  dialectical 168, 169, 217
  enuresis 185
  erectile dysfunction 154
  personality disorders 168, 169
  see also cognitive behavioural therapy
beliefs, abnormal 13
  delusional disorders 92
benzodiazepines 202, 209–11
  acute and transient psychotic
      disorders 96
  agitated/aggressive patients 233
  alcohol withdrawal 230, 231
  anxiety 210–11
    generalised anxiety disorder 125

dementia 41
  insomnia 149, 210, 212
  in pregnancy 160
  schizophrenia acute episode 87
bereavement 122
beta-blockers 202
  generalised anxiety disorder 125
  phobia 129
    social 131
bipolar disorder 115–19, 248(257)
  late-onset 50
  schizoaffective disorder with
      symptoms of 98
birth see perinatal risk factors
blood tests 18
  anorexia nervosa 144
  delirium 37
  delusional disorders 91–2
  dementia 41
  drugs
    mood stabilizers 206, 207
    neuroleptic malignant
        syndrome 225
    overdose 220
  mania 102
  schizoaffective disorder 98–9
  schizophrenia 85–6
  see also full blood count
blues, postpartum 155–6
body dysmorphic disorder 140
borderline personality disorder 163,
    165, 169
brain damage in specific areas 56,
    243(254)
breast-feeding and antipsychotics 201
bromocriptine, neuroleptic malignant
    syndrome 227
bulimia nervosa 145–6
buprenorphine 69
buspirone 125, 211

CAGE questions 8, 62
calcium disturbances 58–9
cannabis 74
  schizophrenia and 79
capacity (mental) 21–2
  assessment 21–2, 239(241)

capacity (mental)(*contd*)
  delirium and 38
  dementia and 41
  electroconvulsive therapy and 213,
      213–14
  fitness to plead and 191
carbamazepine 206, 208, 209
cardiac effects, antidepressant effects 195
cardiovascular examination 17
care coordinator 27
care programme approach (CPA) 27
case summarizing 19
catatonic state
  ECT 261(264)
  in schizophrenia 82
catecholamines, urinary 57, 248(257)
cerebellar damage 56
childhood
  attachment *see* attachment
  depression linked to events in 106
  learning disability and questions
      related to 171
  see also home environment
children 176–88
  hyperkinetic (attention
      deficit–hyperactivity) disorder
      16, 179–80, 252(259)
  patient's 7
  psychiatric assessment 176
  see also adolescents
chlordiazepoxide 68, 230, 231
chlorpromazine, photosensitivity 201,
    263(265)
cholinergic pathway inhibition/
    antagonism *see* anticholinergic
    effects
cholinesterase inhibitors, Alzheimer's
    disease 45
circadian rhythm disorders 148, 149
clinical psychologist 25
closed questions 3
clozapine 80, 85, 199, 204
  side-effects 204, 263(265)
cluster A personality disorders 162,
    163, 164, 168, 169
cluster B personality disorders 163,
    165–6, 168, 169

cluster C personality disorders 163,
    167, 168, 169
cobalamin *see* vitamin B$_{12}$
cocaine 74–5
coeliac disease 253(260)
co-existing disorders *see* comorbid/
    concurrent/coexisting disorders
cognition
  assessment 14, 15, 36
  impairment 16
    in delirium 35
    in dementia 39
    in mania 101
cognitive analytical therapy 168–9
cognitive behavioural therapy (CBT)
  agoraphobia 130
  depression 112
  panic disorder 128
  personality disorders 168
community care 26–7
  team members 25, 26–7
community treatment, supervised 23
comorbid/concurrent/coexisting disorders
  medical disorders and depression 106
  other psychiatric conditions and
    adjustment disorder 137
    anorexia nervosa 142
    depression 106–7
    hyperkinetic disorder 179, 180
    learning disability 173
    somatoform pain disorder 140–1
competence, legal 191
  see also capacity
compulsion 132
compulsory admission *see* hospital
    admission
computed tomography
  Alzheimer's disease 44
  delirium 37
  vascular dementia 46, 47
concentration, assessment 14
concurrent disorders *see* comorbid/
    concurrent/coexisting disorders
conduct disorders 176–8
consciousness, impaired
  in delirium 35
  in substance abuse 71

cortisol and depression 106
couples therapy, depression 112
crack cocaine 75
Creutzfeldt–Jakob disease 53, 54
crime 189–91, 253(260)
    justice system 25
crisis (resolution) team 26, 240(242)
    community care 26
Cushing's disease 57
cyclothymia 120–1

dantrolene in neuroleptic malignant
        syndrome 226
defiant behaviours 178
delirium 33–8
    dementia and delirium vs 36
delirium tremens 229
delusions (and delusional disorders) 13,
        89–92, 244–8(255–7)
    induced 96–7
    in schizophrenia 83, 84
    in substance abuse 71
    types 91, 237–8(240–1)
dementia 38–49
    criminal offences and 191
    depression and delirium vs 36
    general aspects 39–41
    mixed 47
    organic 53–5
    pseudodementia vs 42
demographics (history-taking) 3–4
dependency and dependency
        syndrome 67–8
    alcohol 62–3, 68–9, 70, 231
    opiate/opioid 63, 69–70, 70
dependent personality disorder 163,
        167, 169
depot antipsychotics 205
depression (depressive episodes)
        104–14
    adolescent 185–6, 193
    aetiology 105–7, 113
    anxiety coexisting with 125
    in bereavement 122
    in bipolar affective disorder 115,
        116, 117, 118
    clinical features 107–10, 113–14

differential diagnosis 111
    dementia and delirium 36
    epidemiology 104, 113
    investigations 110–11
    late-onset 51
    management 111–13
    postnatal 156 8
    prognosis 113, 114
    recurrent 113–15
    in schizoaffective disorder 98, 99
    screening for 110
        learning disability and 173
    somatic syndrome and see somatic
        syndrome
desensitization see exposure and
        desensitization
desire (sexual), lack or loss of 151
detention see hospital admission
detoxification
    alcohol 68, 230–1
    opioid 69
development
    history-taking 6
    neurological, and schizophrenia 79
Diagnostic and statistical manual of
        mental disorders see DSM-IV
dialectical behavioural therapy 168,
        169, 217
diet see nutritional and dietary disorders;
        vitamins
differential diagnosis 19, 20
diminished responsibility 191, 253(260)
disulfiram 68
donepezil, Alzheimer's disease 45
dopamine pathways
    antipsychotic effects 200
        side-effects 201
    schizophrenia aetiology 80
Down's syndrome 174
    dementia and 43
dramatic (cluster B) personality disorders
        163, 165–6, 168, 169
drugs (non-therapeutic aspects)
    blood tests see blood tests
    delirium due to 34
    depression due to 111
    history-taking 63–4

drugs (non-therapeutic aspects)(*contd*)
  learning disability due to 170
  overdose 220, 220–1, 238(241)
  recreational *see* substance abuse
  toxicity/toxicology 223–6,
    261–3(264–5)
  screen 86, 125, 251(259)
drugs (psychiatric medication/
    pharmacotherapy) 192–212
  acute and transient psychotic
      disorders 95–6
    postnatal psychosis 159
  agitated/aggressive patients 38,
      231, 233
  alcohol abuse 68
  Alzheimer's disease 45
  bipolar affective disorder 117–18
    late-onset 50
  bulimia nervosa 146
  cyclothymia 120
  delirium 38
  delusional disorders 92
    induced 97
  depression 112
    adolescent 185–6
    postnatal 158
  dysthymia 120
  enuresis 185
  erectile dysfunction 154–5
  generalised anxiety disorder 125,
      212
  history-taking 5
  hyperkinetic disorder 180
  insomnia 149, 210, 212
  learning disability, prescribing 173
  manic episode 103–4
  obsessive–compulsive disorder 134
  opioid abuse 69
  panic disorder 128, 212
  personality disorders 169
  phobias 129
    agoraphobia 130
    social phobia 131
  in pregnancy, prescribing 103, 160,
      201, 207
  premature ejaculation 152
  schizoaffective disorders 99

  schizophrenia 80
  seasonal affective disorder 122
  see also specific (types of) drugs
DSM-IV
  bipolar affective disorder 115
  delusion disorder 90
  depression 109, 110
  personality disorder 163
  schizophrenia 83
DTNBP1 gene 79
dual role trans-sexualism 155
dysmorphophobia 140
dyspareunia 153
dysthymia 119–20, 249(257)
dystonia, acute 227–8, 263(265)
dystrobrevin binding protein 1 gene 79

early intervention in psychosis services
    27, 240(242)
eating disorders 142–6, 252–3(259–68)
ECG 18
ecstasy 74
Edinburgh Postnatal Depression
    Scale 157–8
educational history 6–7
elderly people 49–58
electrocardiogram 18
electroconvulsive therapy 213–15,
    261(264)
  depression 113
    late-onset 51
  manic episode 104
emergencies, psychiatric 218–33,
    261–5
  admission for assessment in 22
emotional numbing, post-traumatic
    stress syndrome 136
empathic statements in interview 3
employment history 7
encephalitis, viral 55
endocrine disorders and hormonal
    abnormalities 56, 57
  depressive episode and 105–6
    differential diagnosis 111
  manic episode in 100, 103
  psychosis in 90
  schizophrenia vs 86

enuresis 184–5
environmental assessment, aggressive/
    agitated patients 232
environmental factors, delirium 34
    see also home environment
environmental management, delirium
    37–8
erectile dysfunction 154–5
erotomanic delusions 91
examination, physical 16–18,
    237–8(240–1)
exhibitionism 156
exposure and desensitization
    in cognitive behavioural
        therapy 216
    obsessive–compulsive
        disorder 134
    phobias 129
        agoraphobia 130
extrapyramidal symptoms
    antipsychotics 38, 50, 87, 95, 160,
        201, 233
    Lewy body dementia 48
eye examination 17
eye movement desensitization and
    reprogramming 136

factitious disorder 141
familial CJD 54
family
    conduct disorders and reporting
        by 177
    interview in child assessment 176
    see also parental factors
family environment see home
    environment
family history-taking (incl. psychiatric
    history) 5–6
    learning disability 173
family studies
    bipolar affective disorder 115
    depression 105
    schizophrenia 78
females, history-taking 7
fetal alcohol syndrome 175
fetishism 156
fitness to plead 191

flooding in cognitive behavioural
    therapy 216
fluoxetine 249(258), 262(264)
    children/adolescents 193
folate deficiency
    alcohol abuse and 247(256)
    Alzheimer's disease and 43
folie à deux 96–7
forensic history 8–9
forensic psychiatry 189–91, 253(260)
formication 229
formulation of case 19
fragile X chromosome 175
frontal lobe lesions 56, 243(254)
frontotemporal dementia 48–9
frotteurism 156
full blood count (FBC)
    delirium 37, 245–6(255)
    schizophrenia 85

GABA
    alcohol and 228, 229
    benzodiazepines and 210
    depression and 105
    non-benzodiazepine hypnotics
        and 211
galantamine, Alzheimer's disease 45
gender identity disorders 155
generalised anxiety disorder 123–5, 212,
    250(258)
genetic factors
    Alzheimer's disease 42–3
    bipolar affective disorder 115, 116
    delusional disorders 89
    generalised anxiety disorder 123
    learning disability 170
    manic episode 100
    obsessive–compulsive disorder 132
    panic disorder 126
    personality disorders 162
    phobias 128
    schizoaffective disorders 97
    schizophrenia 78, 79
    somatization disorder 138
geriatric psychiatry 49–58
glucose, blood 246(256)
glue sniffing 76

grandiose delusions 13, 91, 237(240)
  schizophrenia 84
grief, pathological 122
growth hormone
  depressive episode and 105
  manic episode and 100
guilt delusions, schizophrenia 84
gustatory hallucinations 12
  schizophrenia 84

hallucinations
  in alcohol withdrawal 229
  assessment 11–12
  in mania 101
  in schizophrenia 83, 84
  in substance abuse 71
  visual see visual hallucinations
haloperidol 87
  agitation 38, 231, 233
  neuroleptic malignant syndrome
    with 225, 226
haptic hallucinations 12
harm
  to others/from others, risk 16
  to self see self-harm
  see also abuse
head injury 55
heart see cardiac effects
hebephrenic schizophrenia 81–2,
    247(256–7)
history-taking 3–9, 237–8(240–1)
  synopsis 19
histrionic personality disorder 163,
    166
HIV and AIDS-associated disorders
  dementia 53–4
  psychosis 86
home (family) environment 6
  generalised anxiety disorder and 123
  phobias and 128
  schizophrenia and 80
  somatization disorder and 138
home treatment team 26–7,
    240(242)
homicide
  mood disorder and 190
  schizophrenia and 190

hormonal abnormalities see endocrine
    disorders and hormonal
    abnormalities
hospital admission (compulsory) 22–3
  acute and transient psychotic
    disorders 95
  bipolar affective disorder 117
  delusional disorders 92
  depressive episode 111
  schizoaffective disorders 99
hospital services
  general 26
  psychiatric 26
human immunodeficiency virus
    see HIV
5-hydroxytryptamine see serotonin
hyperactive delirium 35, 36
hyperarousal, post-traumatic stress
    syndrome 136
hypercalcaemia 58–9
hyperkinetic (attention deficit–
    hyperactivity) disorder 16, 179–80,
    252(259)
hypersomnias of central origin 149–50
hyperthyroidism 57, 245(255)
hyperventilation disease and panic
    disorder 126
hypnagogic hallucinations 12
hypnopompic hallucinations 12
hypnotics 209–12
  benzodiazepine see benzodiazepines
  non-benzodiazepine 211
  insomnia 149
hypoactive delirium 35, 36
hypocalcaemia 58
hypochondriacal delusions 91
hypochondriacal disorder 139–40
hypoglycaemia 246(256)
hypomania 102, 115, 116, 118, 121,
    248(257)
hypothyroidism 57

ICD-10
  acute and transient psychotic
    disorders 93–4
  acute intoxication in alcohol/substance
    abuse 64

bipolar affective disorder 116–17
delusional disorders 90
  induced 96
dementia in Pick's disease 48
depressive episode 108
generalised anxiety disorder 123–4
hyperkinetic disorder 179–80
manic episode 101
obsessive–compulsive disorder 133
schizoaffective disorder 98
schizophrenia 80, 83, 83–4
social phobia 131
illusions, assessment 11
induced delusional disorder 96–7
infanticide risk 157, 158
infectious disease
  dementia 53–5
  mania 103
  psychosis 90
injury see abuse; harm; trauma
insanity defence 191
insight 14, 15
  schizophrenia 85
insomnia 147–9, 210, 212,
  253–4(260–1)
International Classification of Diseases
  see ICD-10
interpersonal psychotherapy 216
interviewing
  agitated/aggressive patients 233
  child (with or without family) 176
  techniques 3
  see also questions
investigations 18
  see also specific conditions
involuntary movements 9

jealousy delusions 13, 89, 91, 92, 191

kindling hypothesis, manic episode
  100–1
Korsakoff–Wernicke (amnesic)
  syndrome 60, 71–3

lamotrigine 160, 206, 208, 209
law (and legal issues)
  electroconvulsive therapy and 213–14

mental health 21–3, 238–9(241)
  and criminal offences 191,
    253(260)
substance abuse
  alcohol 63
  legal highs 76
  opiates 64
learning disability 170–5
legal issues see law
Lewy body dementia 47
libido (sexual drive/desire), lack
  or loss of 151
life events, stressful/adverse
  depression and 106
  generalised anxiety disorders and 123
  manic episode and 101
  obsessive–compulsive disorder
    and 132
  panic disorder and 126
  schizophrenia and 80
lifestyle modification
  in opioid abuse 69
  in premenstrual syndrome 161
light therapy, seasonal affective
  disorder 122
lithium 206, 207, 207–9, 223–4
  administration and action 223–4
  bipolar disorder 117
    late-onset 50
  pregnancy and 160
  side-effects and toxicity 207, 208,
    223–4, 238(241), 261(264)
liver function tests (LFTs)
  delirium 37, 245–6(255)
  schizophrenia 85
local authority services 25
lorazepam
  agitated/aggressive patients 233
  schizophrenia acute episode 87
LSD 75, 80
lysergic acid diethylamide (LSD) 75, 80

McNaughton criteria 191
magic mushrooms 75
malingering 141
management plan 20
mania (manic episodes) 100–4

mania (manic episodes)(*contd*)
  in bipolar affective disorder 115, 116,
    117, 118
  criminal offences and 190
  in schizoaffective disorders 98, 99
  see also hypomania
marital status and depression 106
MDMA 74
medical conditions (organic conditions/
    multisystem disorders/physical
    disorders) 56–60
  as cause/risk factor
    delirium 34
    erectile dysfunction 154
    insomnia 147–8
    learning disability 170
    psychosis 90
    sexual loss of desire 151
  as complication
    anorexia nervosa 144–5
    substance misuse 63
  depression and
    concurrent 106
    differential diagnosis 111
  schizophrenia vs 86
  somatization disorder vs 139
medical history, past 5
medication *see* drugs
melancholic depression 109
memantine, Alzheimer's disease 45
memory, assessment 14
  see also amnesia
Mental Capacity Act 21–2
mental health
  assessment *see* assessment
  law 21–3
  substance abuse impacting on 63, 66
    alcohol 63
Mental Health Act 22–3, 239(241)
mental state examination 9–15
mentalization-based therapy 169
metabolic disorders 58
  depression vs 111
  learning disability in 170
  psychosis in 90
methadone 69
methylenedioxymethamphetamine 74

mirtazapine 198
moclobemide 198
monoamine oxidase inhibitor
    (MAOI) 196–7
  mechanism of action 192, 196
  reversible inhibitor of MAO-type A
    (RIMA) 198
monoamine theory
  depressive episode 105
  manic episode 100
mood
  assessment 10–11
  mania and change in 101
  see also affective (mood) disorders
mood stabilizers 117, 118, 206–9,
    261–2(264)
  in pregnancy 160
motivational interviewing, alcohol
    abuse 69
motor and psychomotor disturbances
  in generalised anxiety disorder 124
  in neuroleptic malignant
    syndrome 226
  in substance abuse 71
movements, involuntary 9
multidisciplinary team 24–5,
    239–40(242)
  community care 25, 26–7
  members and their roles 24–5
multi-infarct (vascular) dementia 45–7
multiple sclerosis 60, 243(254)
multisystem disorders *see* medical
    conditions
Munchhausen's syndrome 141
Munchhausen's syndrome by proxy 141

narcissistic personality disorder 163, 166
negative symptoms of schizophrenia 81,
    82, 85, 87
neuroanatomical abnormalities *see*
    neuropathology
neurodevelopmental theory of
    schizophrenia 79
neuroleptic malignant syndrome 201,
    202, 225–7
  see also antipsychotics
neurological disease

depression vs 111
mania in 103
psychosis in 90
schizophrenia vs 86
neurological examination 18
neuronal damage, Alzheimer's
disease 43
neuropathology (incl. neuroanatomy)
Alzheimer's disease 43, 44
obsessive–compulsive disorder 132
delusional disorders 89
Lewy body dementia 47
Pick's disease 48
schizophrenia 80
Wernicke–Korsakoff syndrome 73
neuroses see anxiety and neuroses
neurosyphilis 54–5, 85
neurotransmitter disturbances
delirium 34
depression 105
lithium-related 207
manic episode 100
obsessive–compulsive disorder 132
panic disorder 126
schizophrenia 80
night terrors 150
nihilistic delusions 13, 237(240)
schizophrenia 84
NMDA inhibitors, Alzheimer's
disease 45
non-steroidal anti-inflammatory drugs
(NSAIDs) 246(256)
noradrenergic and specific serotonergic
antidepressant (NaSSA) 198
nurse see psychiatric nurse
nutritional and dietary disorders
59–60
Alzheimer's disease and 43
see also vitamins

obsessions 12, 132
obsessive–compulsive disorder 132–4,
250(258), 252(259–60)
obsessive–compulsive personality
disorder (anankastic PD) 132,
163, 167
occipital lobe damage 56

occupational (employment) history 7
occupational therapist 25
olanzapine 87, 204
old age psychiatry 49–58
olfactory hallucinations 12
schizophrenia 84
omega-3 fatty acids and Alzheimer's
disease 43
open questions 3
opioid/opiate
dependency 63, 69–70, 70
overdose 238(241)
oppositional defiant disorder 178
organic mental disorders 33–61,
243–4(254)
see also medical conditions
orgasmic dysfunction 152
orthostatic (postural) hypotension,
antipsychotics 263(265)
overdose 220, 220–1, 238(240)

Pabrinex 73, 230, 231
pain
in sexual intercourse 153
somatoform pain disorder 140–1
panic attack and disorder 126–8, 212,
238(241), 250(258)
paracetamol overdose 220–1
paranoid (cluster A) personality disorders
162, 163, 164, 168, 169
paranoid schizophrenia 81
parasomnias 150–1
parental factors, conduct disorders 177
see also family
parietal lobe damage 56
Parkinson's disease 38, 47, 100, 105
paroxetine
children/adolescents and 193
pregnancy and 193
passivity phenomenon 14
schizophrenia 85
past history (psychiatric; medical;
surgical) 5
Patient Health Questionnaire (PHQ-9)
110, 111
perception
assessment 11–12, 15

perception(*contd*)
  disturbances
    in delirium 35
    in schizophrenia 83
perinatal (incl. birth) risk factors
  learning disability 171
  schizophrenia 79
persecutory delusions 13, 91, 245(255)
  schizophrenia 84
personal history 6–7
personality
  anorexia nervosa and 142
  generalised anxiety disorder and 123
  obsessive–compulsive disorder
    and 132
  premorbid 8
personality disorders 162–9
  anankastic 132, 163, 167
  criminal offences and 190
phaeochromocytoma 57, 248(257)
pharmacist 25
pharmacotherapy *see* drugs
phenothiazines 200, 201, 203
phobias 12, 128–31
  social 130–1, 250(258)
phosphodiesterase 5 inhibitors, erectile
    dysfunction 154–5
photosensitivity, chlorpromazine 201,
    263(265)
physical disorders *see* medical
    conditions
physical examination 16–18,
    237–8(240–1)
Pick's disease 48–9
piperazine side-chain phenothiazines
    200, 201, 203
planning of management 20
polymorphic psychotic disorder,
    acute
  with symptoms of schizophrenia 94
  without symptoms of schizophrenia 94
positive symptoms of schizophrenia
    81, 82
postnatal disorders 155–60
post-traumatic stress syndrome 135–6,
    249–50(258)
postural abnormalities 9, 18

postural hypotension, antipsychotics
    263(265)
poverty, delusions of 13
pregnancy
  alcohol consumption 175
  assessment with child learning
    disability 171
  drug prescribing in 103, 160, 201, 207
  see also perinatal risk factors; prenatal
    factors
premature ejaculation 152–3
premenstrual syndrome 161
prenatal factors, schizophrenia 79
presenilin genes and Alzheimer's
    disease 43
presenting complaint 3
primary care 26
  panic disorder 128
prion disease 53
procyclidine 38, 202, 233, 263(265)
pseudodementia 42
pseudo-hallucinations 12
psychiatric hospital *see* hospital
psychiatric nurse
  community 25
  inpatient 24, 240(242)
psychiatric services 25–6
psychiatrist, role 24
psychodynamic psychotherapy 216
psychoeducation, cyclothymia 121
psychological therapy (psychotherapy)
    215–17
  acute and transient psychotic
    disorders 95
  alcohol abuse 68, 69
  anorexia nervosa 144
  bipolar disorder 118
  bulimia nervosa 146
  conduct disorder 178
  delusional disorders 92
  depressive episodes 112
    postnatal 158
  erectile dysfunction 154
  generalised anxiety disorder 125
  hypochondriacal disorder 140
  obsessive–compulsive disorder 133–4
  orgasmic dysfunction 152

panic disorder 128
personality disorders 168–9
phobias 129
    agoraphobia 130
    social phobia 131
    post-traumatic stress syndrome 136
    schizoaffective disorders 99
    schizophrenia 87–8
    seasonal affective disorder 122
    somatoform pain disorder 141
psychologist, clinical 25
psychomotor disturbances see motor and
    psychomotor disturbances
psychosexual disorders 151–4
psychosis (and psychotic disorders)
    acute and transient 93–6, 245(255)
    in depression 108, 112
    early intervention services 27,
        240(242)
    in mania, symptoms of 101, 102
    organic conditions causing 90
    postnatal 158–60
    in schizoaffective disorders 98
    in substance abuse 70–1
        residual and late onset 73–4
psychosocial factors
    bipolar affective disorder 116
    conduct disorders 177
    depression 106
    manic episode 101
    self-harm 221
psychostimulants, hyperkinetic
    disorder 180
psychotherapy see psychological therapy
puerperal disorders 155–60
punch drunk syndrome 55
pupils, examination 17

questions
    in interview 3
    screening see screening
quetiapine 204

reactive attachment disorder
    178–9
referential delusions 13, 237(240–1)
    schizophrenia 84

relationships, past and current 7
residual psychosis in substance
    abuse 73–4
residual schizophrenia 82
reversible inhibitor of MAO-type A
    (RIMA) 198
risk assessment 15–16
    forensic patient 189
    self-harm 15, 16, 251–2(259)
risk modification, vascular dementia 46
risperidone 80, 134
    dementia 41
    side-effects 204
    Tourette's syndrome 183
rivastigmine, Alzheimer's disease 45
Russel's sign 146

sadomasochism 156
SADPERSONS mnemonic 219, 220
safeguarding and learning disability
    174
sarcoidosis 61
schizoaffective disorders 97–9
schizoid personality disorder 163,
    164
schizophrenia 77–88, 190, 244–8
    (255–7)
    acute polymorphic psychotic
        disorder with or without
        symptoms of 94
    aetiology 78–80, 88
    clinical features 80–4
    crime and 189, 190
    epidemiology 77–8
    investigations 85–6
    late-onset 49–50
    management 86–7
    prognosis 88
    screening for 84–5
        learning disability and 173
schizophrenia-like psychotic disorder,
    acute 94, 245(255)
schizotypal personality disorder 163,
    164, 169
Schneider's first-rank symptoms 83
schoolteachers, conduct disorder
    reporting 177

screening (incl. questions)
  acute stress reaction 135
  adjustment disorder 137
  delirium 35–6
  dementia 40
    Alzheimer's disease 44
    vascular dementia 46
  depression see depression
  generalised anxiety disorder 124
  insomnia 148
  learning disability 171
  obsessive–compulsive disorder 133
  phobias 129
    agoraphobia 130
    social phobia 131
  post-traumatic stress syndrome 136
  premature ejaculation 152
  schizophrenia see schizophrenia
  self-harm 15, 222–3
  suicide 218–19
seasonal affective disorder 121–2
secretary 25
seizure threshold in ECT 214
selective serotonin re-uptake inhibitors
    (SSRIs) 194–5
  bulimia nervosa 146
  first-line use 193
  generalised anxiety disorder 125, 212
  late-onset depression 51
  mechanism of action 192
  obsessive–compulsive disorder 134
  panic disorder 128, 212
self-harm 221–3, 251–2(259)
  adolescent 186–7
  risk assessment 15, 16, 251–2(259)
self-help 25
  panic disorder 128
self-neglect 16
septic screen, delirium 37
serotonin (5-hydroxytryptamine;
    5-HT)
  panic disorder and 126
  schizophrenia and 80
  see also noradrenergic and specific
    serotonergic antidepressant;
    selective serotonin re-uptake
    inhibitors

serotonin–noradrenaline re-uptake
    inhibitors (SNRIs) 198
  mechanism of action 192, 198
serotonin syndrome 196
sexual dysfunction 151–4
skin signs/marks/scars, examination
    for 17
sleep cycle (and sleep–wake cycle) 147
  disturbances (=sleep disorders)
    147–51, 253–4(260–1)
    delirium and 35
    depression and 107
sleep hygiene 149, 254(260)
social factors see psychosocial factors
social function disorders, child 178–9
  see also antisocial personality disorder
social history 7
social impact
  alcohol abuse 63
  opiates 64
  schizophrenia 78
social phobia 130–1, 250(258)
social worker 25
solvent abuse 76
somatic syndrome
  depression with 108, 109, 113, 117,
    249(258)
  depression without 109, 113, 117,
    248(257)
somatization disorder 138–9
somatoform autonomic dysfunction
    140
somatoform pain disorder 140–1
somnambulism 150–1
specialist teams in community
    care 26–7
speech assessment 9–10, 15
stress see acute stress reaction; adjustment
    disorder; life events; post-traumatic
    stress syndrome
substance abuse 62–76, 244(254–5)
  acute intoxication 64–6
  adolescent 187–8
  affective disorders 71, 103
  harmful use 66–7
  history-taking 8, 62–4
  insomnia in 148

mania in 103
  older people 53
  urine drug screen 246(255)
suicide 218–21, 251–2(259)
  adolescent 186–7
  older people 52
sulpiride 201
  Tourette's syndrome 183
summation (summarizing)
  after interview 3
  of case 19
supervised community
    treatment 23
surgical history, past 5
symptoms
  in history-taking 4
  in mental state examination 9–15
  see also specific disorders
syphilis, neurological 54–5, 85
systemic lupus erythematosus 60

tactile hallucinations 12
tangentiality 249(257)
tardive dyskinesia 263(265)
teachers, conduct disorder
    reporting 177
team see multidisciplinary team
temporal lobe damage 56
thought alienation (delusions with
    regard to possession of
    thoughts) 14
  schizophrenia 83, 84
thought content 12, 15
thought disorders (generally) 12
  formal 10, 15
thought echo 83, 84
thyroid disorders/dysfunction (incl.
    thyroid hormone abnormalities) 57,
    245(255)
  depressive episode 106
  manic episode 100
  schizophrenia 85
  tests of thyroid function 37, 85,
    250(258)
tics 183
Tourette's syndrome 183
toxicology see drugs

transvestism, dual-role 155
trauma/injury
  head 55
  learning disability 170
  see also abuse; harm
treatment 192–217, 261–5
  admission for 22
  supervised community 23
tricyclic antidepressants 195–6
  anticholinergic effects 195,
    262–3(265)
  mechanism of action 192, 194
twin studies
  bipolar affective disorder 115
  depressive episode 105
  manic episode 100
  schizophrenia 78, 79
tyramine and monoamine oxidase
    inhibitors 197

urea and electrolytes (U&E)
    247(256)
  delirium 246
urinary tests 18
  catecholamines 57, 248(257)
  drug screen 246(255)

vaginismus 153–4
valproate/valproic acid 206, 207,
    208, 209
  bipolar disorder 117, 118
vascular dementia 45–7
vascular disease, psychosis 90
venlafaxine 198, 262(264)
viral encephalitis 55
visual hallucinations 11, 247(256)
  mania 101
  schizophrenia 84
vitamin(s) (in general), deficiencies
  mania 103
  psychosis 90
  see also Pabrinex
vitamin B_{12} (cobalamin) deficiency
    59–60
  alcohol abuse and 247(256)
  Alzheimer's disease and 43
  psychosis due to 86

vitamin C and Alzheimer's
    disease 43
vitamin E and Alzheimer's disease 43
voluntary hospital patient, compulsory
    detention 22–3
voyeurism 156

Wernicke–Korsakoff (amnesic)
    syndrome 60, 71–3
Wilson's disease 59, 243–4

withdrawal state, alcohol 67, 228–31,
    244(255)
women, history-taking 7

Yale–Brown Obsessive–Compulsive
    Scale 133

z-drugs (non-benzodiazepine
    hypnotics) 211